NEUROANATOMY
SIMPLIFIED

Additional Publications by the Author
Which May Be of Interest to Rehabilitation Personnel

1. J.C. Moore, "Neuroanatomical and Neurophysiological Factors Basic to the Use of Neuromuscular Facilitation Techniques" Pp 31-85, 10 illust. In: Occupational Therapy for the Multiply Handicapped Child. Editor: W. West. Published by University of Illinois, 1965. 338 pp.
2. J.C. Moore, "The Developing Nervous System in Relationship to Techniques in Treating Physical Dysfunction." Chapter 1 in Expanding Dimensions in Rehabilitation. Pp. 3-20 Editor: L. Zamir, C.C. Thomas, 1969.
3. J.C. Moore, "Structure and Function of the Nervous System in Relation to Treatment Techniques." Chapter 2 in Expanding Dimensions in Rehabilitation, Pp. 21-41. Editor: L. Zamir, C.C. Thomas, 1969.
4. J.C. Moore, "Confusion and Controversy Concerning Treatment Techniques Utilized in Physical Dysfunction." Chapter 3 Editor: L. Zamir in Expanding Dimensions in Rehabilitation. Pp. 42-51. C.C. Thomas, 1969.
5. J.C. Moore, "Perceptual-Motor Dysfunction in Rehabilitation Personnel. Editorial. AJOT Jan.-Feb. 1966. Vol. XX, No 1, Pp. VII, 46-47.
6. J.C. Moore, "Changing Methods in the Treatment of Physical Disfunction." AJOT Jan.-Feb. 1967, Vol. XXI, No 1, Pp. 18-28.
7. J.C. Moore, "Basic Research in Occupational Therapy." In Proceedings of the Occupational and Physical Therapy Conference on Research, Puerto Rico, 1967. Published by Department of Health, Education and Welfare, Washington, D.C., 1967.

NEUROANATOMY
SIMPLIFIED

SOME BASIC CONCEPTS FOR UNDERSTANDING
REHABILITATION TECHNIQUES

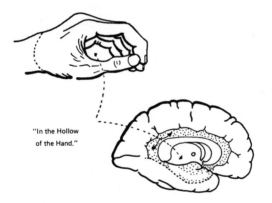

"In the Hollow
of the Hand."

Josephine C. Moore, OTR, PhD

*University of South Dakota
Medical School*

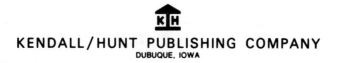

KENDALL/HUNT PUBLISHING COMPANY
DUBUQUE, IOWA

To my father and mother,

Professor and Mrs. A.D. Moore

Contents

Foreword

During the past several years, occupational therapy has undergone much investigation, evaluation and reorganization with the intended result of stimulating and implementing professional growth and strength. Since "the whole is the sum of its parts," the profession can progress only proportionately to the professional growth of the individual members. "Continuing education" is a necessity for all O.T.R.s to retain, to gain or to regain information vital to professional proficiency. This article is one of a planned series of presentations by its author and provides one tool with which clinicians, teachers and investigators can better equip themselves to make a more knowledgeable contribution to patient treatment in all fields of occupational therapy.

Lyla M. Spelbring OTR, MA

Preface

Many rehabilitation therapists today find themselves in a rather peculiar situation concerning the newer rehabilitation techniques, especially the concepts underlying these techniques. The words neuroanatomy and neurophysiology, proprioceptive neuromuscular facilitation, perceptual motor dysfunction, facilitation, inhibition etc., cause one to wonder if he will ever be able to comprehend this vast area of information. This article is an attempt to help therapists "bridge the gap" in their knowledge and perhaps establish a basic foundation upon which they can build additional information.

One has to admit that neuroanatomy and physiology are not simple. However, if one desires to grasp the basic fundamentals, he must begin someplace. That "someplace" is memorizing essential terms, structures, pathways and connections. Many of us fail to understand an area of knowledge because we dislike memorizing facts or claim that we "cannot memorize things." Yet we go through life committing to memory names of friends, vital statistics such as the amount of a pay check, deductions, prices of food, clothing, birth dates, anniversaries etc. We even, without realizing it, can tell a person how to travel from one place to another over complicated routes through cities, countryside and even through the modern highway clover-leafs or interchanges. Road travel today is much more complicated than the pathways, connections and routes of the nervous system that a therapist should know. Therefore, if we are capable of learning geography, we should be able to learn the fundamental concepts of the nervous system. Once these basics are committed to memory, we can travel the side pathways and smaller towns along the way and slowly build up an interchange system which will take us in any direction we wish in order to obtain a desired result. That which follows has been purposely kept on a very simple level. It may insult some readers (for whom it is not intended) but it may stimulate others to memorize the basic building blocks concerned with the understanding of neuroanatomy and neurophysiology.

Chapter I

Basic Concepts and the Spinal Cord

THE CENTRAL NERVOUS SYSTEM

We shall begin with neuroanatomy, which merely means the structure of the nervous system. The function, or neurophysiology, will be discussed at a later time.

Man has divided the nervous system into two fundamental parts— that which is *central* and lies within a bony protective covering and that which is *peripheral* and lies outside of this bony structure. However, man's division is a false one, since the two parts are so interconnected that one cannot function normally without the other. Therefore we will try to think in terms of one complete nervous system, realizing however that the two parts are necessary for discussion purposes. We can say that the central nervous system is like a large department store, with the peripheral nervous system being the outlying countryside or area around the store with roads and/or streets leading into and out of this area (Figure 1).

If we think of the central area as a large department store (Figures 1 and 2) with many levels, we can discuss each floor as a separate yet combined part of the total structure. Our store has 37 levels. These levels are connected by stairways, escalators and express elevators. We also have to imagine that *every* level has entrances and exists from the outside.

Thirty-one of these levels (representing the spinal cord segments) sell only basic merchandise. The thirty-second level (the first part of the brain stem or *medulla* has machinery in it for automatic control of the escalators, elevators, heating plant, water system etc., as well

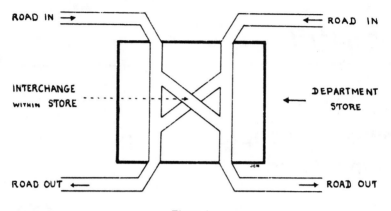

Figure 1.

as being a connecting link between lower and higher levels. The thirty-third level (*Pons*, or "bridge" portion of the second part of the brain stem) is in interchange center for routing information between lower and higher levels and to the big computer system which is housed, like a cantilever structure, over the thirty-second, thirty-third, and thirty-fourth levels. (This is the cerebellum, or "little brain," the thirty-fifth level, Figure 2.) The thirty-fourth level (uppermost part or third part of the brain stem, or *midbrain*) has offices which relay information up and/or down to other levels, receives information from the computer on the thirty-fifth level (cerebellum) and runs other vital systems which will be discussed later. The thirty-sixth level (subcortical gray, or deep gray area under the cerebral cortex), known as the *diencephalon*—meaning "throughbrain or between-brain"—is of utmost importance. Almost all information must be processed through this center in order that things run smoothly and a constant check and balance be kept in the entire store. It has very close connections with the computer in the thirty-fifth level (cerebellum) as well as higher and lower levels.

The last or thirty-seventh level is the penthouse (*cerebrum*, meaning brain, or *telencephalon*, meaning "tel" = operating at a distance, + enchephalon + brain. The word *tele*phone utilizes this prefix and means communication at a distnace). Here in the telencephalon the top executives control all other levels, except for those affairs which can be controlled by management at lower levels. Here too, memory of past events is believed to be stored and referred to when necessary. Here the store profits or loses in the competitive market.

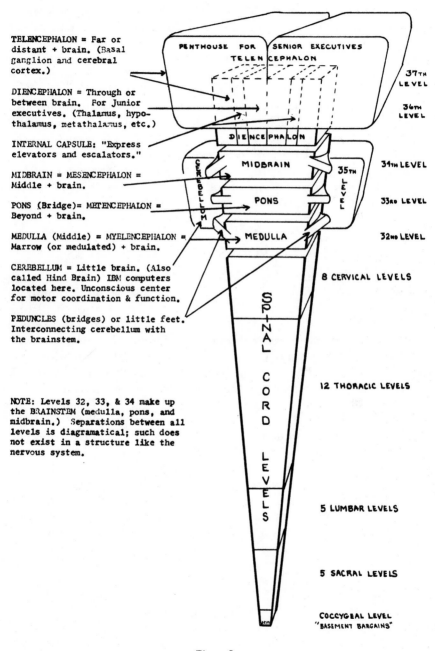

TELENCEPHALON = Far or distant + brain. (Basal ganglion and cerebral cortex.)

DIENCEPHALON = Through or between brain. For Junior executives. (Thalamus, hypothalamus, metathalamus, etc.)

INTERNAL CAPSULE: "Express elevators and escalators."

MIDBRAIN = MESENCEPHALON = Middle + brain.

PONS (Bridge)= METENCEPHALON = Beyond + brain.

MEDULLA (Middle) = MYELENCEPHALON = Marrow (or medulated) + brain.

CEREBELLUM = Little brain. (Also called Hind Brain) IBM computers located here. Unconscious center for motor coordination & function.

PEDUNCLES (bridges) or little feet. Interconnecting cerebellum with the brainstem.

NOTE: Levels 32, 33, & 34 make up the BRAINSTEM (medulla, pons, and midbrain.) Separations between all levels is diagramatical; such does not exist in a structure like the nervous system.

PENTHOUSE FOR SENIOR EXECUTIVES TELENCEPHALON

37TH LEVEL

36TH LEVEL

DIENCEPHALON

CEREBELLUM

MIDBRAIN

35TH LEVEL

34TH LEVEL

PONS

33RD LEVEL

MEDULLA

32ND LEVEL

8 CERVICAL LEVELS

SPINAL CORD LEVELS

12 THORACIC LEVELS

5 LUMBAR LEVELS

5 SACRAL LEVELS

COCCYGEAL LEVEL "BASEMENT BARGAINS"

Figure 2.

The entire 37 levels must function as a total entity. Breakdown or malfunction of one part affects the whole. Therefore, no part can be divorced from another. The entire structure and contents act as a coordinated nervous system to run things smoothly (Figure 2).

In spite of the central store being complete within itself, it is worthless unless customers purchase merchandise. Therefore, perhaps the most vital part of the store is its periphery—the surrounding area which links it with the outside world—equivalent to the peripheral nervous system. Eliminate all incoming customers (stimuli) and the store is valueless. Death of business results. Stimuli from the periphery *must come first* with response (or purchase of goods) last.

In summary, we can say: demand = supply or stimulus = response. This dare not be expressed in reverse order for the nervous system does not operate in that manner, nor does business.

CENTRAL NERVOUS SYSTEM CONNECTIONS

Before proceeding, the reader should have gained some basic knowledge concerning the nervous system and should commit to memory those technical terms of the various hierarchies of the "store levels" in Figure 2. Each term has been broken down into prefixes and suffixes, making it easier to understand how and why these levels are named. In this way one automatically learns the functional sequence of the nervous system, from lowest levels to highest, as well as their basic purposes in the hierarchy of running a nervous system. Also, one obtains a fundamental concept of the development (phylogeny) of the nervous system that has gone on for millions of years. This developmental sequence began with simple spinal creatures and evolved up through the invertebrates and vertebrates, including man.

Earlier, we stated that stairways, escalators and express elevators connected our store levels with one another. The stairways connect one level with the next. The escalators also connect one level with the next but only go in one direction—either up or down. The express elevators skip many floors and only stop at certain prescribed levels. They also go up (or down), i.e., they carry messages only in one direction like the escalators. In the early days when our store was first built, it had only stairways.

As time passed (evolution), one-way escalators were installed to speed up service between customer and management. At the same time, it was decided that to avoid congestion of traffic in and out of the store only the back doors would be used for entering the structure and the front doors for leaving the building (Figures 1 and 3).

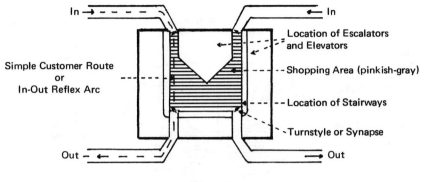

In

In

Location of Escalators
and Elevators

Simple Customer Route
or
In-Out Reflex Arc

Shopping Area (pinkish-gray)

Location of Stairways

Turnstyle or Synapse

Out

Out

Figure 3.

Still later, one-way-up and one-way-down express elevators were installed to expedite messages and help coordinate all areas of management. Long since, the computer was placed on the thirty-fifth cantilevered floor (Figure 2) for coordinating all business that did not have to reach junior or top executive levels for major decisions. Now our store was complete, just so long as the customers (stimuli) continued to demand the supplies and carry them out of the store.

Let us look at the basic floor plan of level 17 as an example (Figure 3). Our customer enters a rear store door and has to pass through a turn-style (synapse: syn = together,—aps = joining) before being allowed to shop. The shopping area is all painted a pinkish-gray, so that the customer can tell at a glance those areas where sales items and sales personnel (cell bodies) can be contacted. To the periphery of the gray area are white areas. That white area closest to the gray area is where the stairs are located. Beyond are the one-way escalators and one-way express elevators (pathways or tracts) (Figure 3 and 4).

If a customer desires to obtain one item on floor level 17, he locates it and purchases it from a saleslady (synapses with a cell body) then leaves through a turnstyle (synapse) out of the front door. This is a simple function or a simple reflex arc. However, our customer decides to shop around. He walks up the peripheral white stairs to level 18 or he can choose to go down to level 16. From here he can exit or continue up or down. He can, if in a hurry, take an escalator up or down, or better yet, an express elevator. However, these express elevators are only for customers (our stimuli or impulses) who must converse with the higher levels, such as bill-paying,

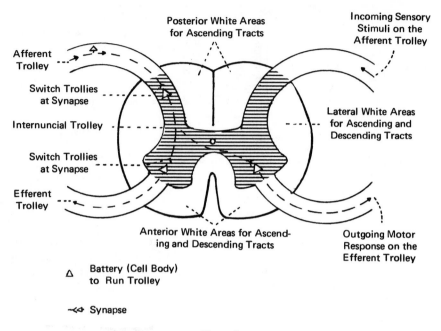

Figure 4.

straightening out an account, better service demands etc. Therefore, many impulses entering the store can be handled on lower levels and they can exit from these lower levels. But complaints, bills, purchase slips, inventory of items sold, replacement of items purchased, running the store, etc. must be sent up to higher levels to be registered, scrutinized and acted upon to keep things running smoothly. Also, any ideas the junior or top executives have that will assist the customer in any way can be sent down to lower levels via the stairs (slow handling of items and business), or down escalators (faster management) or via "down" express elevators for speedy expedition of service needs.

As business increases management has to devise a way to control the tremendous influx of impulses (customers), purchases and messages going hither and yon. A decision is made whereby every customer travels on a little trolley to gain entrance into the store, to shop around and to leave the store. The *afferent* trolley ("going toward") carries them into the store (Figure 3). Once in the back door they must synapse (switch or make connections) with an inter-trolley (the internuncial neuron or interneuron) if they plan to shop on just that floor. Leaving they must take the _efferent_ ("going away") trolley out of the store.

If one desires to go upstairs or down, he must either switch to a stairs trolley, escalator trolley or express elevator trolley. In some cases, however, the accommodations are such that one can remain on his afferent trolley and go up (or down) for quite a way before having to switch trolleys on a higher or lower level. Management has also decreed that for certain items of business the customer must use certain prescribed facilities (up or down elevators, escalators etc.) for gaining the floor level on which he wishes to do business. If he wishes to deal in feelings (tactile sensations), vibrations or conscious position senses, he must use the posterior column white areas to gain a higher level. Should he have a pain, he must use a lateral white column pathway. If he is having thermostat problems (temperature), he will utilize the same elevators or escalators used for those who have pain. Many more examples could be cited. However this suffices to show how specific management has become in order to cope with the demands of business (stimuli) and attempt to coordinate and satisfy every specific area so that things can be run efficiently.

In summary: The gray area of each floor level is for customer use and sales contacts (location of cell bodies in the spinal cord) which are confined to each specific floor level. The white areas are for either up (or down) connections between adjacent floor levels and/or a floor level with much higher (or lower) centers. We now have our basic cross sectional floor pattern, or architecture, of the nervous system as concerns level 1 through 31. We can also add here that, in general, the two sides of the store (or nervous system) are bilaterially symmetrical or mirror images of one another. Therefore only one-half of the floor plan need be labeled or learned.

CROSS SECTION: SPINAL CORD

With this information we can add to the basic floor plan of levels 1 through 31, as diagrammed in Figure 5.

Up until Figure 5, everything was progressing rather well for the reader. Here, however, a long sigh is heard and the words . . . "Oh no, not again!" Yes, again and again and again. We must go over these floor plans and learn them in order to understand what comes next.

One should try to commit to memory everything up until now. Right here is where most of us have trouble. We hope in some vague and yet unknown way that we will be able to understand these newer rehabilitation techniques without learning the basic concepts con-

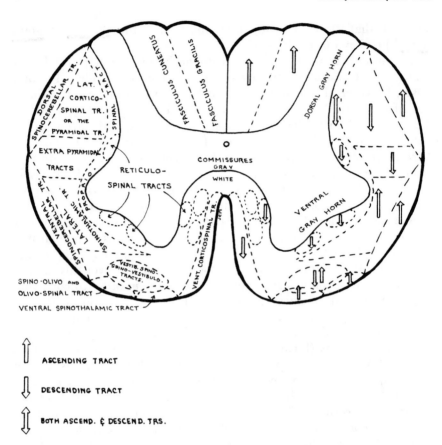

ASCENDING TRACT

DESCENDING TRACT

BOTH ASCEND. & DESCEND. TRS.

Figure 5.

cerning the structure and function which underlie them. We now stand at the crossroads of decision. We can learn now in order to understand what follows or admit that we lack the discipline necessary to help ourselves learn. If we begin learning today, tomorrow we can help others. The decision is our own. No one else can learn it for us.

TERMINOLOGY

Before completing this ara of knowledge, we should obtain a basic understanding of those simple words—*sensory* and *motor*. Sensory implies the perception or perceiving of a stimulus. When we smell something burning, we are perceiving a stimulus. The odor which reaches our special senses (smell) tells us something. How we interpret the odor depends upon past experiences stored in higher levels of the nervous system. We react to the stimulus by doing something and this reaction is a *motor* response to a simple stimulus. Notice that the stimulus has to preceed the motor response, not vice versa.

The nervous system has three ways of perceiving sensations. First: It can pick up sensations from our external skin surface (touch, tactile, temperature, pain etc.) or via our special senses (seeing, hearing, smelling, taste or equilibrium) and react to any *changes* which these systems perceive. Those stimuli which are picked up by receptors "outside of us" are called *exteroceptors*, meaning exterior receptors which are near our skin (cutaneous sensation) or heard, seen, smelled, etc. Thus, the exteroceptors are a group of general and specialized receptors which receive stimuli from the periphery of our bodies. One should note that receptors only react to *change*, an important point to remember.

Second: We have stimuli which come from the inside of our body and are picked up by receptors called *interoceptors* (received from the interior). These tell us we are hungry, nauseated, cold, hot, in pain etc. These can also be referred to as visceral receptors or receptors of visceral stimuli.

Third: We have receptors concerned with movement and posture. These receptors are neither internal (visceral) nor external (skin and special senses) but lie in an intermediate position, around joints and ligaments, in muscles and tendons, in the pads of our hands and feet and in our inner ear. There are also specialized receptors which are associated with muscle tendons, joints, fasicia, etc. These are called *proprioceptors*, i.e., receptors of "one's own." (Proprius (L) = one's own.) The word "property" is from this same latin word. Certainly among the greatest properties man has are the muscles and tendons which endow him with the ability to move, communicate, express ideas, create and survive. One can argue that our intellectual capacity is our greatest asset when compared with other animals. However, this is of no value unless we have the means whereby to carry out our thoughts, ideas and feelings. Without muscle and proprioceptive sensation from muscle and allied structures, we cannot write, speak intelligently, see or hear normally or communicate in any known way. Therefore, perhaps our greatest endowment is our property to move and to use this movement effectively to carry out the necessities of life.

Muscle for movement's sake is valueless however unless we somehow know at all times what a muscle is doing. In order for muscle to work smoothly, maintain posture and position sense, move, lift, walk, shove, etc., we must have a sensory mechanism which initially perceives a stimulus as well as a sensory "feedback system" from our muscles, tendons, ligaments etc., to tell us what is going on at every moment. This is what our proprioceptors are for. They send sensations to the nervous system to keep it continually informed so that we can use the muscle or muscle groups as needed. Unless these proprioceptors are intact, our muscles are, for all essential purposes, of little or no value to us.

In summary: First, we need a sensory stimulation to activate the nervous system. In turn, the nervous system reacts by moving muscle. This reaction is the *motor* response to the stimulus. That impulse (stimulus) which comes in the "back door" of the spinal column (or higher levels) is the trigger which sets into motion some recordable response and movement results. It cannot work in reverse, i.e., motor first, stimulus last. All movement, therefore, is the motor result of some preceeding stimuli. Or simply, stop all stimuli from occurring and the result is lack of movement—a nothingness . . . death.

Chapter II

Introduction to the Neuron

INTRODUCTION

Chapter I of this series introduced to the reader a general concept of the nervous system. It attempted to relate the following ideas: (1) Why the nervous system is important in order to understand how man functions, (2) the "divisions" of the nervous system and their "hierarchy" of development and function, (3) a basic understanding of the gray and white matter of the spinal cord and the concept of stimulus-response mechanisms and (4) some basic concepts of terminology that should be understood before delving further into this area of knowledge.

The next three chapters will deal with the *neuron*. One might ask "Why is this single nerve cell so important? Why can't one learn more about the total nervous system and how it relates to rehabilitation principles, instead of studying neurons?" Simply stated, if one fails to understand the basic parts of a system and how they function, one cannot adequately comprehend how the total system functions. The "total is the sum of its parts" and this principle holds when discussing any subject no matter how simple or complex it may be. Wouldn't one understand the conflict in Viet Nam better if one were well versed in the historical events leading up to the present? Would not the civil rights issue be clearer to us if we had lived 150 years ago or 100 years ago both as a Negro and white? More basically, wouldn't therapists have a much greater faith in their profession and better understand their role in medicine if they understood all of the facts, concepts and principles which make up our body of knowledge? This author believes so. In like manner, one can gain a much broader comprehension of neuroanatomy and neurophysiology if one first understands the smallest functioning part of the nervous system—the neuron. The neuron is the *fundamental structure* of the nervous system. Over 20 billion of these microscopic cells act to coordinate, integrate and ultimately run all of the other systems of the body, thus making man the unique creature that he is.

THE NEURON

Man, as an organism, operates in two environments. One environment is that of the organism itself, i.e., the total body consisting of skin, heart, lungs, digestive system, emotions, actions, hormones, nerves, health, etc. The other environment is that which surrounds him, i.e., temperature, humidity, air, light, home, people, work, play and other psychosocial phenomena. The organism, in some way, must attempt to maintain a balance (homeostasis) between the internal environment and its needs and that of the external environment and the demands which it places upon it. In order to balance these forces, the organism must have some way of perceiving stimuli so that it may cope with both the internal and external demands. We know of only one way in which this can be accomplished and this is the utilization of the neurons which comprise the nervous system.

The principle function of a neuron is, first, to receive stimuli; second, to conduct or transmit these stimuli or impulses along the neuron; and last, to pass this information to other structures in the organism. These impulses can be received from either the external environment (exteroceptive stimuli) or the internal environment (proprioceptive and interoceptive stimuli). Next, they are transmitted from neuron to neuron or to non-nervous cells of the body, such as muscles, glands, etc., (Figure 6).

These billions of neurons are responsible for coordinating all bodily functions, such as circulation, respiration, stress, movement, thinking, emotions, interactions with others, etc. Without neurons, we would have no connecting links between the many systems of our body and the outside environment. Therefore, the total organism is dependent upon neurons to keep it operating efficiently and normally, thus maintaining equilibrium or homeostasis. Unbalance this system, damange it or place excessive stress upon it and we see instead a pathological reaction, i.e., mental illness, general malaise, hyper- or hypotonicity, incoordination, tachycardia, temulence, fibrillation, thanatomania, etc.

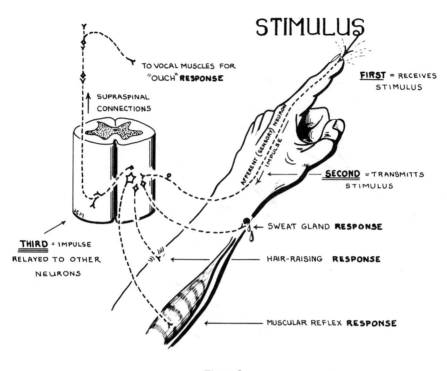

STIMULUS

FIRST = RECEIVES STIMULUS

TO VOCAL MUSCLES FOR "OUCH" **RESPONSE**

SUPRASPINAL CONNECTIONS

AFFERENT (SENSORY) NEURON IMPULSE

SECOND = TRANSMITTS STIMULUS

← SWEAT GLAND **RESPONSE**

THIRD = IMPULSE RELAYED TO OTHER NEURONS

HAIR-RAISING **RESPONSE**

MUSCULAR REFLEX **RESPONSE**

Figure 6.

The Fundamental Parts of the Neuron

The classical definition of a neuron is "a nerve cell body and all of its processes." A neuron, whether it is unipolar (having one major process or pole extending from the cell body), bipolar (having two major processes) or multipolar (having many processes) (Figure 7), has one cell body. From this a number of branches or processes extend for varying distances. These processes have been given specific names: (1) Dendrites (dendron = tree; dendrites = branches of the tree) or processes which conduct impulses *toward* (afferent) the cell body, (2) axon or axis cylinder (axon = central core, branch, or process) which conducts impulses *away* (efferent) from a cell body or (3) a peripheral process conducting *toward* the cell and a central process conducting *away from* the cell body (Figure 7). At the termi-

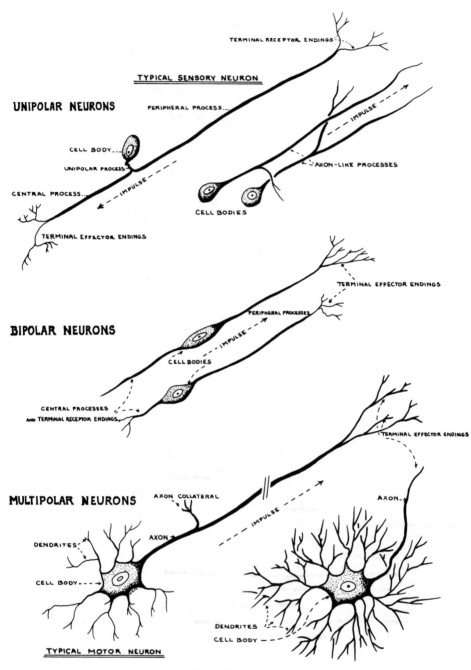

Figure 7.

nation of these processes we find specialized types of endings. These are for receiving stimuli and/or passing these impulses on to the next neuron or to non-nervous tissue. (Specialized receptor endings will not be discussed at this time.) One can understand neurons and their processes if we liken a neuron to a car battery (Figure 8). The battery is equivalent to the cell body of a neuron. Inside the battery are

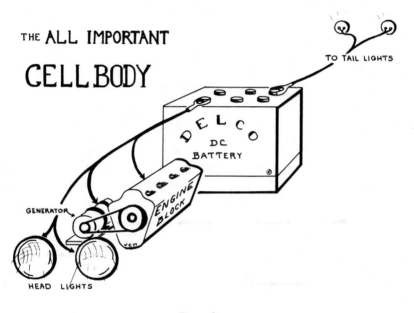

Figure 8.

chemicals and plates which generate electro-chemical responses. As long as the battery is in good condition it is alive and can function to turn the car on, operate head lights, radio, windshield wipers, etc. In order for the battery to run these various parts there must be a connection between the battery and the part. This connecting wire is equivalent to a neuronal process extending from the cell body. It may be short or it may be extremely long, such as the wire extending from the battery to the tail lights.

As long as the battery remains in good condition, as well as the wires extending from it, the car runs properly. Let the battery go dry or become cracked and chances are that it will die. Its processes, however, may still be intact and unharmed. But these processes can no longer carry electrical impulses, for the cell body (battery) has ceased to function. We can purchase a new battery and make the car operate again. This is not true in the nervous system. When a cell body dies, the processes extending from it eventually die. In time, even other nerve cells connected with it or non-nervous cell connections that are controlled by this neuron die. To preserve the integrity of a neuron, all of its parts and the structures associated with it, it must be functioning normally in order for the neuron to receive and transmit stimuli.

Terminology

Before taking up the various kinds of neurons found in the nervous system, it would be best to clarify some terminology. The meaning of the word "innervation" should be examined. Some have the idea that this term applies only to the effector end of a neuron i.e., where a motor neuron effects or innervates muscle. However, the receptor end of a neuron is also spoken of as innervating a structure.

The skin is innervated by sensory neurons, viscera is innervated by neurons of the autonomic nervous system and muscle is innervated by proprioceptive fibers which pick up sensory impulses from the muscle. Therefore, when the term "innervation" is used, it implies either the effector (efferent) or receptor (afferent) part of the neuron and the structure with which it is associated. In like manner, a neuron interposed between two other neurons (an interneuron) is innervated by the neuron or neurons which synapse upon it. Therefore, the term "innervation" is a general one implying the distribution of a neuron (or neurons) to any structure, whether it be another neuron or non-nervous tissue. More simply stated, it means to "supply with nerves" (Webster).

Another area of possible confusion arises when we speak about a *neuron* versus a *nerve*. Technically, a neuron is a single cell body with all of its processes. A nerve is made up of hundreds of neurons grouped together in a common connective tissue sheath. Some authors prefer to differentiate these two terms by stating that a neuron is a microscopic structure while a nerve consists of many neurons and is a structure that is large enough to see with the naked eye. In spite of these defined differences, these two terms are not always used correctly. Frequently one finds that the term "nerve" is substituted for, or used interchangeably with, the word "neuron." Therefore, it behooves the reader to not only know the correct definitions of these two words but also to understand that these terms can be used as synonyms. Rarely is the term neuron substituted for nerve but frequently the words nerve and neuron are used to describe the same structure, i.e., a neuron or single nerve cell and all of its processes.

Kinds of Neurons

In the nervous system there are many "kinds" of neurons, such as association neurons, internuncial neurons, projection neurons, commissural neurons, sensory neurons, bipolar, unipolar, Betz cells, Purkinje cells, Alpha and Gamma motoneurons, Golgi Type I and II, Group Ia or Ib, or Group II neurons, etc. (It would seem that man has had a delightful time trying to systematize and categorize the various types of neurons found in the nervous system. Specific names are very helpful when discussing in depth neurons and their functions. However, they are quite confusing to the individual attempting to gain a basic understanding of neuroanatomy.) For practical purposes we can speak of just three kinds of neurons: (1) Sensory neurons, (2) motoneurons and (3) interneurons (also called internuncial or intercalated neurons) (Figure 7). The interneuron is not specifically a motor or a sensory neuron. Rather, it serves as a vital connecting link between various sensory and motor neurons (Figure 9). Like motor and sensory neurons, however, it still has a similar structure and function. Many of the neurons illustrated in Figure 7 function as interneurons whether they be unipolar, bipolar or multipolar in structure.

Sensory neurons like all other neurons have a cell body (Figure 7). From this cell body (or perikaryon) extend two distinct elongations. These processes tend to resemble one another, i.e., they look alike or appear like an axon. In the normal functioning nervous system an impulse can travel in one direction only, that is, from the receptor ending to the effector ending, not vice versa. Stated more simply, the impulse usually travels from a more peripherally located area to a more centrally located structure. With sensory neurons the impulse traveling from the receptor ending first traverses the peripheral or afferent process (afferent = going toward the cell body) and then the central or efferent process (efferent = going away from) (Figure 7).

Motoneurons have many short dendritic branches sprouting directly from the cell body and one longer process extending from it (Figure 7). The smaller and finer dendritic branches, as well as the cell body, act as receptors (afferent processes). The large single process (which may be quite long in comparison to the dendrites) is the effector (efferent process) or axon. Again, like all neurons in the nervous system the impulse can travel in only one direction, i.e.,

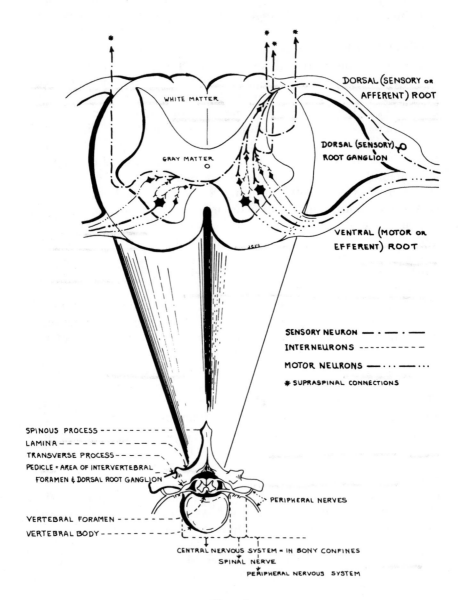

Figure 9.

from receptor to effector, not vice versa. Motoneurons like sensory neurons are found both in the central and peripheral nervous systems (Figure 9). However, the cell bodies of these two types of neurons are always located within the central nervous system (that is, within the bony confines of the vertebral column or the skull). Their processes, however, can either be confined within the central nervous system or can extend beyond its confines to make up the peripheral nervous system. (An exception to this general rule is found in the autonomic nervous system. "Half" of the cell body population of this system is located within and the other "half" outside of the central nervous system.)

Interneurons (internuncial neurons) serve as connections or neuronal bridges between sensory and motor neurons. They have receptor (afferent) and effector (efferent) processes, as well as a cell body. They are located entirely within the confines of the central nervous system (Figure 9). Interneurons cannot be classified as truly sensory or motor neurons. For now, we shall consider them as connecting links between the sensory and motor systems. More recent thoughts concerning these interneurons put them in a rather unique category. It is theorized that the major integrative and coordinative functions of the nervous system take place in the interneuronal nerve cells.

For a long time textbooks, instructors and clinicians have placed the major emphasis of nervous functioning upon the motor side of the nervous system. This was a natural "error" as one can *see* and record this system much more readily than the sensory system. The emphasis is now shifting to the sensory side. We are becoming more and more aware of the vital role of sensory receptors in helping the organism cope with the internal and external environment. Also, we are aware that the motor system appears to be almost completely subservient to the demands placed upon it by the sensory system.

Now we must adjust our focus even finer. We must look to the connecting links (interneurons) found between these two systems in order to better understand how the total system functions. It is here that we may find our answers to the way in which the nervous system adapts, summates, facilitates, inhibits, coordinates and integrates all of the information constantly bombarding it. These interneurons are found in great numbers in such important structures as the thalamus, basal ganglion, cortex, corpus callosum, supra- and intra-spinal connections and the all important reticular system to mention a few.

In summary, it behooves the reader to think of the *motoneuron* as the last link in a chain of commands (Figure 10). This neuron represents the non-commissioned officer who carries out all the orders of

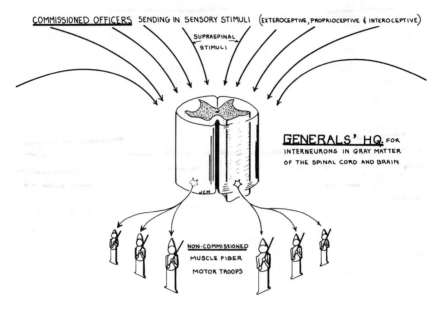

Figure 10.

the higher command. That is not to imply that the motoneuron is unimportant. Rather, it is to impress the reader with the idea that it is useless unless it receives well "thought out" orders and carries them through like a well-mannered servant or robot. Once ordered, it can do nothing but carry out the demand placed upon it.

The *sensory neuron* could be equated to a commissioned officer somewhere in the ranks from lieutenant to colonel (Figure 10). Its vital role is to be aware of every stimulus coming to the organism from both within and without. It is theorized that this officer has the ability to modulate and/or ignore subthreshold stimuli but it must pass on all information of threshold value into the system. Without these sensory command officers the system is helpless. The organism cannot function at all even though all of the non-commissioned "motor troops" exist in full force. In like manner, if one deprives these sensory officers of receiving information, or in reverse, bombards them with too much information (stress), the nervous system begins to break down and malfunctioning occurs.

This could be equated to an all out rout, retreat or mass confusion in the system. It can no longer properly judge incoming impulses or handle the volume of information "attacking it" (or lack of volume in the case of sensory deprivation). This also leaves the non-commissioned "motor officers" in a helpless state. They either have no reliable officer to give them meaningful orders, no orders at all or the orders which are received are so confused that they become meaningless. The result may be catastrophic.

Last, but not least, are the *interneurons or the* vital connecting links between the sensory system and the subservient motor system (Figure 10). These neurons should probably have the rank of general. It is this rank that will have past events stored within it. Therefore, it can modify messages coming into it from the sensory officers and also judge what messages should be passed on. It is this command post which filters out unnecessary information. It relays only that which is most important to the survival and maintenance of the total system. Otherwise, it is the integrative system of the organism. It is the most vital component which is responsible for seeing to it that homeostasis is maintained and that appropriate action is carried out to achieve this result.

THE SYNAPSE

At the "interval" between two neurons, whether it is between a sensory and motoneuron, a sensory and interneuron or an interneuron and motoneuron, we find a microscopic gap or space (Figure 11). This gap is called the *synapse* (syn = joining, apse = together). Here the impulse is relayed from one neuron to the next at a speed of about 0.6 milliseconds (one-half of a thousandths of a second). Where a motoneuron connects with non-nervous tissue, such as a muscle, we use a different term. This can be called a junction, such as the myo-neural junction (muscle-nerve junction), motor end plate, end foot or simply termination (Figure 12). In other words, when neuron meets neuron we have a synapse. When neuron meets non-nervous tissue we have a junction.

At these synaptic or junctional locations one finds an electro-chemical reaction taking place which either serves to help (facilitate or excitate) or hinder (inhibit) the transference of the impulse across the gap. It is not necessary to delve into the biochemical and electrical phenomena which occur within these structures. A few basic

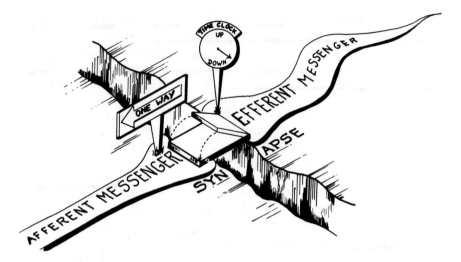

Figure 11.

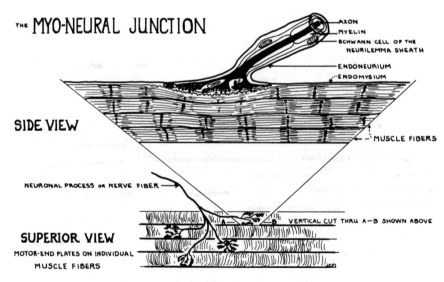

Figure 12.

principles should help us understand how an impulse is transmitted from one structure to the next or prohibited from crossing this area. For an analogy, we can think of a drawbridge which crosses a moat (Figure 11). This drawbridge is quite different from those seen during the days of King Arthur. This is a modern bridge—so modern in fact that it only accepts one-way traffic. Traffic flow is such that the "messenger-impulse" can travel only from the efferent road, (or axon of one neuron), over the bridge to the afferent road (or dendrite) of the next neuron. This assures the system that no messages can travel backwards and mess up the normal functioning of stimuli coming in and motor going out.

When the drawbridge is down, the stimulus messenger can cross over and make contact with the opposite side (with either another sensory neuron in the chain, an interneuron or a motoneuron). When the drawbridge is up, no impulse can cross over. Therefore, our bridge has two special features or mechanisms built into it. First, passage is unidirectional, i.e., from axon to dendrite (of another cell) or efferent to afferent. The second feature is a time clock or lock like those found in a bank vault. This timing mechanism allows the bridge to stay down for only a specific length of time before the bridge automatically raises itself again. This prevents the bridge from being left open. It also allows it to "rest" and prepare itself for the next messenger-impulse.

The biochemical molecules located at synapses act in a similar manner. The electrical impulse coming along the neuronal process to the bridge travels unidirectionally. When this reaches the gap, it causes the release of a chemical substance which flows across the gap and contacts the opposite bank, thus letting down the bridge (Figure 11). This activates the neuron that is waiting on the other side or the non-nervous tissue which may be next in line for receiving this impulse. As soon as this occurs, a second chemical is released. This inactivates the first chemical that was released into the gap or raises the bridge. This second chemical prohibits another message from "crossing over" until the original chemical "rebuilds itself" to threshold strength. Once back to full power it can be reactivated by the next impulse coming down the neuronal process.

Unfortunately, one cannot generalize and state that chemical "A" always lowers all bridges in the body or that chemical "B" raises them. The nervous system is not that simple. In the millions of years over which it evolved, different kinds of chemicals were utilized for the control of various systems in the body. Today, we find some drawbridges that function by using one set of bio-chemical bridgelowerers or bridge-raisers while at another gap we find a different set operating.

It is not within the scope of this paper to delve into the biochemistry of these different kinds of synapses. Rather, it is hoped that one obtains a general concept, i.e., in order to transfer an impulse from one neuron to another or to non-nervous tissue it must cross a microscopic gap. This gap has unidirectional properties just as do neuronal processes. When the impulse reaches the gap, an electro-chemical response occurs. This allows the impulse to cross over, in a very brief span of time, before an inhibitor chemical "closes" the gap again.

Chapter III

The Neuron (Continued)

CONDUCTION VELOCITY AND INSULATION
OF NEURONAL PROCESSES

Cell bodies of neurons come in all sizes and shapes (Figure 13). Neuronal processes also have a variety of configurations, varying lengths and diameters. We have neurons whose axon diameters are extremely thin or small. Others have intermediate to large axonal diameters. The diameter of the neuronal processes helps to determine the conduction velocity for that neuron. Conduction velocity indicates the rate or speed of transmission of an impulse as it travels along the neuronal process. The general rule to follow is that the larger the axon diameter or neuronal process (Figure 14) the faster the impulse travels and vice versa.

Most processes of neurons (either their peripheral or central processes, axons or dendrites) have an insulating-like-substance covering them. This material which we call myelin (myelin = marrow or white fatty material) (Figure 15 and 16). It can be equated to the insulation seen on telephone cables or household wiring. In an ordinary house wire one finds two copper lines running within a common sheath (Figure 15). If one examines these wires carefully, he finds that the wires are separated from one another by some kind of insulating material. This prevents the wires from coming into contact and causing a short circuit or "cross-talk" between adjacent wires. In like manner, neuronal processes are insulated from neighboring processes to prevent cross talk or short circuiting in the nervous system. In any home one also finds many kinds of insulated wires. Some are very thinly insulated like those carrying electricity to a lamp. Others have a heavier coating (or several wrappings) of insulation such as the

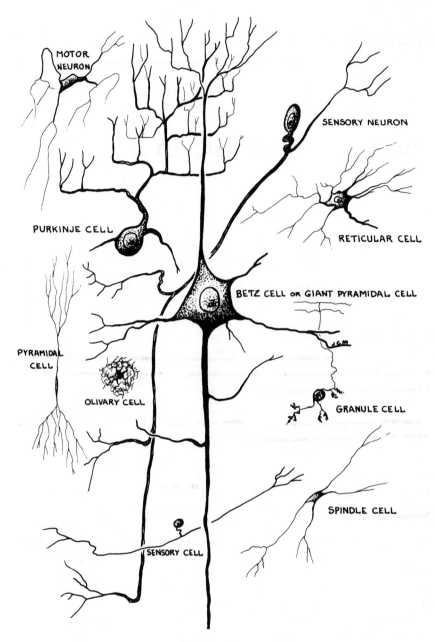

Figure 13.

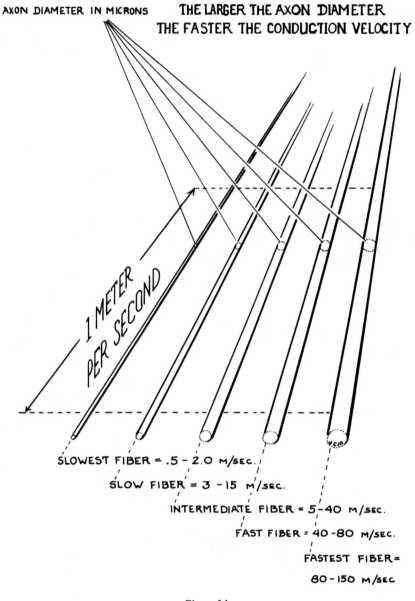

AXON DIAMETER IN MICRONS

THE LARGER THE AXON DIAMETER
THE FASTER THE CONDUCTION VELOCITY

1 METER PER SECOND

SLOWEST FIBER = .5 - 2.0 M/SEC.

SLOW FIBER = 3 - 15 M/SEC.

INTERMEDIATE FIBER = 5 - 40 M/SEC.

FAST FIBER = 40 - 80 M/SEC.

FASTEST FIBER = 80 - 150 M/SEC

Figure 14.

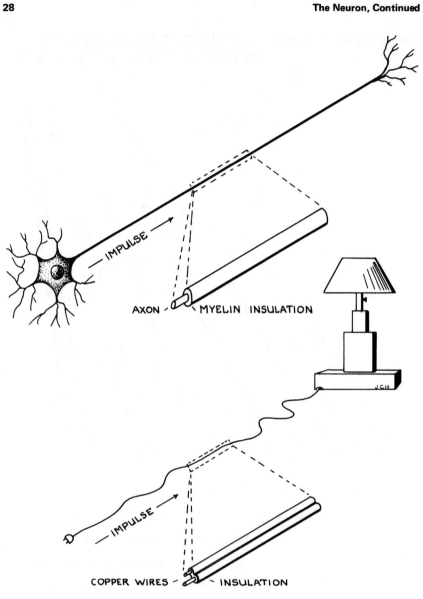

IMPULSE

AXON   MYELIN INSULATION

IMPULSE

COPPER WIRES   INSULATION

Figure 15.

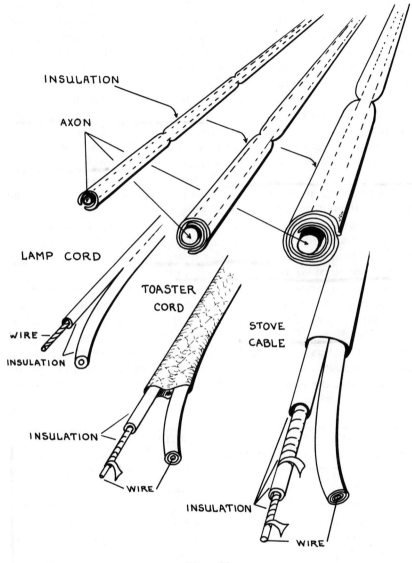

INSULATION

AXON

LAMP CORD

WIRE

INSULATION

TOASTER CORD

STOVE CABLE

INSULATION

WIRE

INSULATION

WIRE

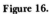

Figure 16.

electrical cable to the stove or refrigerator (Figure 16). Intermediate types of wires service toasters, mixers and similar appliances. Careful examination of the actual wires found within the insulating material shows us that some wires are more delicate or fine (lamp cord) while others are thicker or heavier (cable to a stove).

In the nervous system we find thick neuronal processes which have a very heavy coating of insulating material or myelin. We speak of these neuronal processes as being heavily myelinated (or medullated). With very thin delicate neuronal processes the insulation is similar, i.e., a very minimal amount of myelin is found around the process. We speak of these neuronal processes as being thinly myelinated (medullated) or "non-myelinated"). In the nervous system we find many gradations in diameters of neural processes, as well as the amount of insulation covering them (Figure 16).

The amount of myelin covering neuronal processes is another factor which helps determine the conduction velocity for the neuron. Generally speaking, the heavier the insulation (or myelination) the faster the speed of conduction of an impulse (Figure 16).

In the human nervous system there are about four or five different recognized speeds (conduction velocities) for nerve impulses traveling along neurons (See Chart 1). The speed at which an impulse travels is measured in *Meters Per Second.* In man this can vary from as high as 120 to 175 meters per second (m/sec) and sometimes greater down to about .5 m/sec, depending upon the kind of fiber stimulated, its axon diameter, the amount of insulating myelin covering it and some

AXON DIAMETER IN MICRONS (μ)	CONDUCTION VELOCITY IN METERS PER SECOND	GENERAL FUNCTION
12 - 20 μ	80 - 150 m/sec	PROPRIOCEPTION AND MOTOR
8 - 12 μ	40 - 80 m/sec	TOUCH
1 - 8 μ	5 - 40 m/sec	PAIN AND TEMPERATURE
3 μ	3 - 15 m/sec	AUTONOMIC NEURONS PRE-GANGLIONIC FIBERS
1 OR LESS μ	0.5 - 2.0 m/sec	AUTONOMIC NEURONS POST-GANGLIONIC FIBERS

Chart 1.

other factors which shall be considered later. Slower conducting neurons are usually concerned with autonomic or involuntary functions such as digestion, respiration, etc. Faster neurons are concerned with voluntary or conscious functions such as sensory receptors or motor neurons for muscle movement. Exceptions to this will be discussed later. For now, it is sufficient to remember that we need faster neurons for voluntary or conscious acts and slower ones for unconscious or involuntary (autonomic) responses.

When the myelin covering of a neuronal process was discussed, the nerve sheath which secretes the myelin was purposely not mentioned. This sheath, called the Schwann cell sheath (after Schwann, a German anatomist and physiologist, 1810-1882) or neurilemma sheath (neuri = nerve, lemma = husk or covering) is found only outside of the central nervous system (CNS). That is, it exists only in the peripheral nervous system (PNS) (See also Figure 9, Chapter II, section A). We speak of this sheath (which is believed to be responsible for making myelin) as either the *Neurilemma Sheath*, Schwann cell sheath or the sheath of Schwann (Figure 16). This covering or husk actually wraps itself around the neuronal process like a jelly roll wrapped around a central core (Figure 17). The core represents a neuronal process; the jelly, the myelin; and the bread of our jelly roll, the neurilemma sheath. However, in a jelly roll one notices that the jelly has soaked into or become an intricate part of the bread. In like manner the "myelin" and the "neurilemma sheath" are inseparable. Thus, the myelin is not a separate entity but rather part of the neurilemma sheath.

Because of older terminology and ideas which are still present in the literature, we refer to the inner coils of the neurilemma sheath as the myelinated area while only the outer most coil is referred to as the neurilemma sheath (Figure 17). If one were to place a great number of jelly rolls end to end leaving a microscopic gap between each two but allowing the central core to continue unbroken through each roll, then one would have a structure very similar to a heavily myelinated neuron with its neurilemma sheath. An unmyelinated neuron would have very little to almost no "jelly roll" around it though it would still have the "bread" or neurilemma sheath (Figures 16 and 17).

The neurilemma sheath is believed to be responsible in part for nerve regeneration. If a peripheral nerve is cut and then properly sutured, we may get nerve regeneration. The central core will regrow down the neurilemma sheath and attempt to reestablish contact with the structure(s) it once innervated. (Regeneration growth rate is from

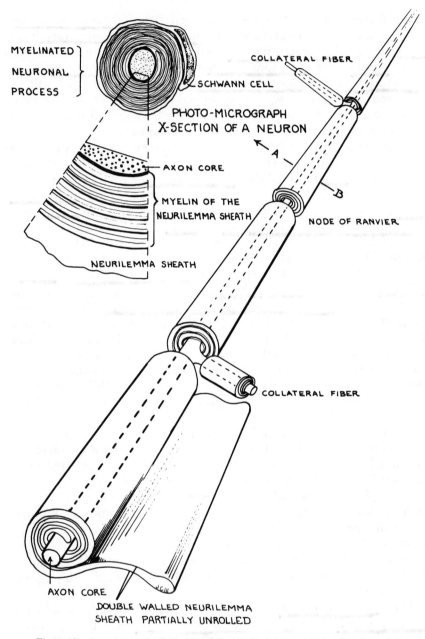

Figure 17. *Concept:* Jelly Rolls Placed End to End Around Unbroken Axonal Core.

one to four millimeters per day, depending upon where the nerve is cut, which nerve is cut, and the conditions of the area through which it is growing.)

Central nervous system neurons lack neurilemma sheaths. (These neurons are myelinated or "unmyelinated." The sheaths, however, come from a different kind of nervous tissue, i.e., glial cells or more specifically oligodendroglia. For some unknown reason, these sheaths either do not have regenerative capacity like that of the neurilemma sheaths in the PNS or some other factor or factors prohibit nerve regeneration in the CNS. For the sake of simplicity, we can say that nerve regeneration is impossible in the CNS (except under well-controlled experimental conditions on subhuman animals). In man's PNS nerve regeneration is fairly successful. But one must remember, however, that if the cell body of a damaged neuron dies, the entire neuron dies.

Nodes of Ranvier and Their Importance

Referring to Figure 17 and our jelly roll concept, we see microscopic gaps existing between each jelly roll. These are called nodes of Ranvier. (Ranvier, a French pathologist, 1835-1922, wrote about these areas and they were subsequently named after him.) Actually, a node is defined as a "knot or swelling along a structure" (Webster). Here, it describes a constricture or gap between two somewhat swollen sections of the neurilemma sheath. The importance of this structural gap is twofold. First, at these gaps one finds collateral nerve processes or branches coming off from the main nerve axon (Figures 13, 17 and 18). Often we think of a neuron as resembling a small section of a non-access highway. This is a misconception. Instead we should understand that most neurons have numerous branchings or collateral fibers extending at right angles from the main axonal process (Figures 13, 17 and 18). This enables one neuron to communicate (synapse) with many other neurons. Consider a non-access "highway neuron." It could be limited to receiving one impulse at a time through a single entry gate. It could transmit only this one impulse down its single non-access highway. Upon leaving a single exit gate it could synapse with perhaps only one or two other non-access neuronal highways. This would give us a one to one ratio of neuron to neuron and would prove to be quite cumbersome, making for an extremely bulky nervous system.

Instead we have highways or neuronal processes that have numerous side roads. These side roads connect with literally hundreds of other neurons and may even send branches back to their own cell

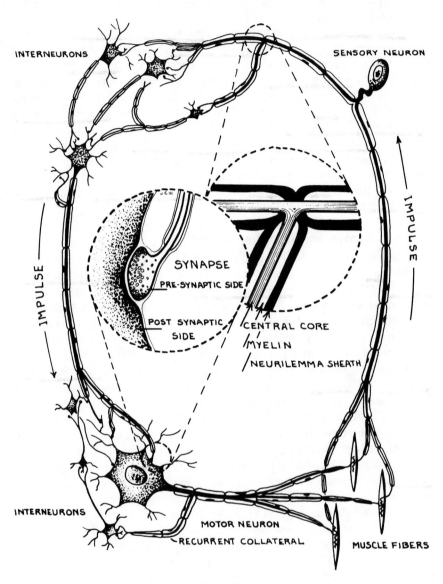

Figure 18.

bodies as self-regulating mechanisms (Figure 18). This may not make for simplicity in understanding the nervous system but it does make for excellent communication among the many and varied parts of the nervous system. It also enables many more areas of the nervous system to be knowledgeable about what is going on in other areas. One neuron can send its impulse (information) to many others simply via its collateral branches which synapse on many adjacent nerve cells or neuronal processes. (The cells of the cerebellum are an excellent example and can readily be used to demonstrate this concept. In fact, the term "avalanche conduction" has been used to express this idea when speaking of cerebellar input and output. It should remind one of the dangers involved in rolling just one little stone down a steep embankment (Figure 19). This one pebble is capable of knocking several others loose upon first impact and, in turn, these knock more loose until an avalanche of formidable magnitude is obtained.) If one remembers this, then he can better conceptualize the nervous system and how it can or may respond to just one impulse or stimulus. This may be great enough to set into motion many reactions, both conscious and unconscious, i.e., a single stimulus can create a tremendous response. This is a well-known phenomenon in psychiatry and in behavioral studies of humans to certain situations. Unfortunately, it is too often forgotten when one deals with the intricacies of the nervous system.

It is with this collateral system and the use of interneurons that we can bombard other cells with information and make them fire more easily (facilitate or excite them) or actually prevent them from firing by inhibiting them. In other words, we need a system whereby we have a spread of information from one cell to many (Figure 18). This plays a vital role in enabling us to have a well-run and smoothly coordinated nervous system.

The second major function of the nodes of Ranvier is concerned with the conduction velocity of neurons. The neurophysiological factors involved in this are too extensive to enumerate here. One can still understand the basic concepts concerning nervous system functioning without delving into the biochemical and electrical phenomena concerned with transmission of nerve impulses. It is sufficient to state that the nodes of Ranvier play a part in the spread of the impulse along neuronal processes. One can equate this type of conduction to an ordinary sidewalk. This sidewalk is like those we see everywhere with expansion joints or "cracks" appropriately spaced between each section (Figure 20a). If one were to walk down this sidewalk, one's pace would be moderate to slow—just a normal

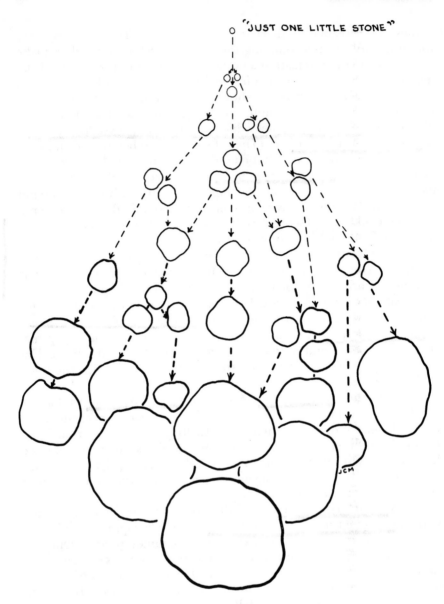

Figure 19. Concept of Avalanche Conduction.

saunter. If instructed to step only on the cracks, one would find himself leaping from crack to crack and traveling the length of the walk at a very rapid pace. This is known as *Saltation,* i.e., "the act of leaping" (Dorland's) (Figure 20a). In the nervous system it is actually transmitted by leaping from node to node (Figure 20b).

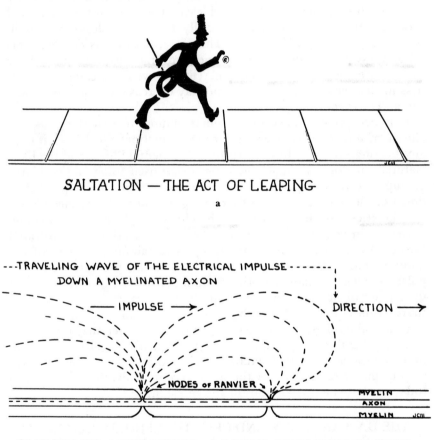

SALTATION — THE ACT OF LEAPING

a

SALTATORY CONDUCTION — LEAPING FROM NODE TO NODE

b

Figure 20.

When this is found, it is also postulated that less myelin is necessary, i.e., with the addition of nodes to the system we can decrease the amount of insulation needed. Earlier it was stated that the greater the amount of myelin the faster the nerve impulse traveled along the neuronal process. In time, the need for increased speed, requiring increased myelination, could add a great deal of bulky covering to neuronal processes and leave little room for the neuronal processes themselves. This is especially true if we desire to obtain speeds up to 120 to 175 m/sec. Therefore, nature has designed this saltatory system whereby she can speed up transmission yet not have to increase the amount of myelin. This allows for greater compactness in the nervous system yet in no way decreases conduction velocity but enhances it.

Is it necessary to have some understanding of such things as myelination, nodes of Ranvier, saltatory conduction, etc.? Does it have any bearing on rehabilitation techniques, mental illness and the like? Naturally it does. Many of the drugs being used today in psychiatry act upon different parts of the nervous system and help to slow down or block transmission of incoming stimuli or act to speed it up. Cryokinetics (the use of ice) in rehabilitation, physical training and surgery is in vogue today. Cooling (as well as heating) has profound effects on the nervous system and upon metabolic processes of the body. Cooling effects a change on the transmission rate of an impulse, as well as changing other functional states (known as, "after discharge" of nervous impulses). In disease, such as hyper- or hypothyroidism, conduction velocity is modified to such an extent that it is measurable. This knowledge is giving us another diagnostic tool and may further help explain one individual's sluggishness or another's hyperactiveness. Therefore, a little knowledge in this area will help us understand some of the more recent innovations being used today in medicine, rehabilitation and research.

THE DAM ANALOGY AND CELL THRESHOLD CONCEPTS

Another concept that we should understand concerns the *threshold* of nerve cells. This can best be explained by the analogy of a body of water that is dammed up. If we wish to maintain the water level at a certain height, we do so by keeping it dammed up at this prescribed level. Let us assume that we desire to hold the level at 70 feet above sea level (Figure 21). This maintained water level can be called the resting level or "resting potential." That is, we have a *potential* source of water which is available to us should we desire to

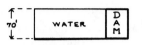 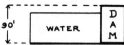 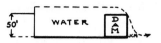

RESTING POTENTIAL   FLOW INHIBITED   FLOW FACILITATED
MAINTAINED THRESHOLD   INCREASED THRESHOLD   DECREASED THRESHOLD

Figure 21. The Dam Analogy.

use it to generate electricity by allowing this water to flow over the dam. Thus, the threshold or resting potential of our lake is held constant at 70 feet above sea level. If we wish to change the threshold from its resting potential, we can either lower the dam allowing the water to flow or we can raise it and prevent it from flowing (Figure 21).

This concept can be applied to the resting potential of a neuron. In the resting state of a neuron (when it is not transmitting an impulse), it has a "resting potential" of about negative 70 millivolts (−70mv) or negative 70 thousandths of a volt potential. In order for the nerve cell to fire (transmit an impulse), this resting potential must be changed, i.e., lowered toward zero (Figure 22). Once it is lowered to a certain critical level (about −50mv), it automatically fires or transmits its impulse. In like manner, we can increase the threshold by raising the dam. The threshold now has a greater nega-

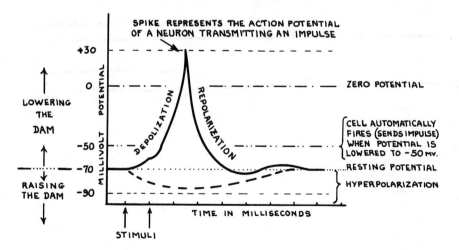

Figure 22.

tive millivolt potential. This might be −75mv, −90mv or even −100mv. This makes it harder to fire the cell as the cell must reach −50mv in order to respond to a stimulus and transmit that impulse. Therefore, if we raise the threshold, it now takes more than just 20 millivolts to change its threshold to the firing level of −50mv. In other words, in its resting state, it only took 20mv to get it to fire—which is a much easier task than when the resting potential is raised.

We can state that the higher we raise the dam (increasing the threshold) the harder it is for water to flow. We are, thus, *impeding* or *inhibiting* its flow or preventing the cell from being able to fire as readily (Figure 21). By lowering the dam we facilitate or make it easier for water to flow. Actually, there are many more factors involved. However, this serves to give us an understanding of the threshold concept of a nerve cell body, as well as a method for changing the cell's potential or its ability to be fired.

It is postulated that facilitation and inhibition of neurons in the central nervous system are accomplished in one of several ways. There may be cells that are only inhibitory in nature, i.e., they can only inhibit other cells from firing by raising their thresholds. Other cells may be only facilitory in nature. Or there may be "inhibitory chemicals" at certain synapses, while at other synapses (on the same cell) we may find only "excitatory or facilitory chemicals." Or a combination of these may occur, plus many more factors which we need not concern ourselves with at the moment.

Whatever the case, we do know that a single cell body in the nervous system is capable of being both facilitated and inhibited (or having its threshold regulated) by other cell processes synapsing upon it. In fact, it is postulated that as many as two thousand to ten thousand or more synapses can be found upon one cell body and its processes (Figure 23). All of the cells synapsing upon a single nerve cell can influence that cell by changing its threshold, i.e., raising or lowering its dam, preventing or assisting it in sending an impulse out over its axonal process.

In summary, we can say that if the balance of synaptic impulses reaching a cell is in favor of inhibiting that cell (i.e., more neurons reach the cell which are inhibitory in nature or carry inhibitory influences), then we cause the cell threshold to be raised (raising the dam) and, thus, prevent the cell from firing. Contrarily, we can bombard a neuron with "facilitatory impulses" and lower the dam, thus, decreasing the electrical potential or threshold of the cell to the −50mv level and allow it to fire (Figures 21 and 22). This gives us

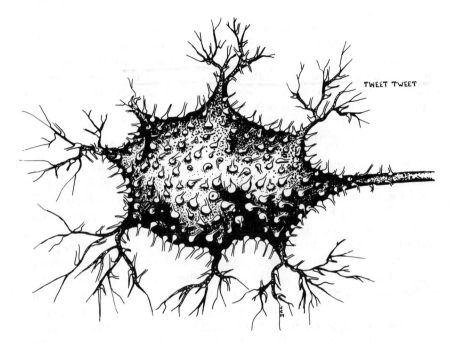

TWEET TWEET

Figure 23.

one of the major concepts of how the nervous system works. It is a check and balance or a facilitation-inhibition system. We can postulate that for every neuron or group of neurons acting to facilitate another neuron there are probably an equal number that also inhibit that neuron. In this way we keep each and every nerve cell in a balanced state, preventing it from firing all of the time yet allowing it to fire when needed.

A simple example of these principles can be illustrated by considering the action of two muscle antagonists. If we desire to contract only our biceps brachii muscle, we facilitate those cells which are resonsible for causing these muscle fibers to contract. At the same time, we inhibit cells that would cause contraction of the triceps brachii. This enables the triceps fibers to relax or give way to movement of the contracting biceps. However, we do not wish to go around all day with the biceps contracted. When we are through with the desired action we relax the biceps by inhibiting the very cells which originally were facilitated during contraction. Naturally it is not this simple but this serves to acquaint us with the elementary functions of nervous system control over just one neuron or over billions. It is this basic principle which allows us to function as well-coordinated organisms. Pathological conditions interrupt this check and balance or facilitation-inhibition system. Hence, we see incoordination, weakness, dissociation of a personality, hypo- or hypertonia, psychosis, neurosis, etc.

FEEDBACK OR SERVOMECHANISMS

The above concept alone will not give us a coordinated system unless we add to it a feedback mechanism. This is vital for it is the way in which each nerve or group of nerves (nuclear groups) can be informed of: (1) What *has just taken* place, (2) what *is taking* place at the moment and (3) what *may take* place in the next millisecond. Initially, we have only discussed three kinds of neurons: the sensory, the motor and the interneuron and their collaterals (See Chapter II, The Neuron). These very same kinds of fibers are also involved in this mechanism which enables the nervous system to know at all times what is going on throughout the entire organism. In Figure 24a we show only a simple chain of neurons. This would be a very primitive type of nervous system. Probably such a system is no longer represented in man. In Figure 24b and 18 we have added a feedback mechanism or servomechanism. (Servomechanism is defined as an

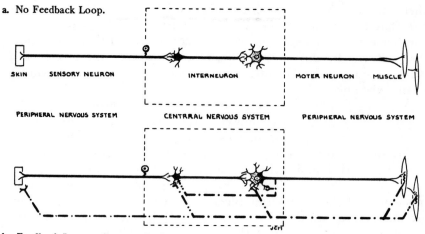

a. No Feedback Loop.

SKIN   SENSORY NEURON   INTERNEURON   MOTER NEURON   MUSCLE

PERIPHERAL NERVOUS SYSTEM   CENTRRAL NERVOUS SYSTEM   PERIPHERAL NERVOUS SYSTEM

b. Feedback Loop or Servomechanism.

Figure 24.

"automatic device for controlling large amounts of power by means of very small amounts of power which automatically corrects performance of a mechanism" (Webster). This servomechanism or feedback loop is essential to all nervous system functioning. Collateral fibers, interneurons (or similar fibers with many names of their own), sensory and motor fibers serve to send information around the nervous system so that all parts are constantly informed in one way or another concerning what is going on (Figure 18). These servo-fibers can come from or belong to exteroceptive, proprioceptive and/or interceptive fibers.

This type of servomechanism might be compared to several nations who are all competing in a space race. Each nation is working separately yet all are cooperating with one another to achieve the best possible result and eventually reach the moon. In order to assist one another, lines of communication are set up between nations. Receiving and sending devices which monitor every space capsule ejected into the atmosphere are also monitored by every nation (Figure 25). In this way one can obtain information either from or to the space vehicle (representing the PNS), as well as from every nation involved in the project (representing the CNS). This illustrates feedback principles in that everything that is going on is known by all, including the space ship zooming towards the moon.

Figure 25 also enables us to understand another concept which applies to nervous system functioning. This deals with injury and the resultant compensatory routes which the system has for handling insult. If we cut the lines of communication between nations A and B, we temporarily lose contact between these two parties. Contact can be reestablished by simply re-routing our information channels from A to C then C to B. However, with the space capsule (representative of the peripheral nervous system), once feedback is lost it can be a rather serious problem trying to reestablish communication again, unless we can go out into space and somehow re-suture the feedback lines.

All of this, of course, is simplified, for we are dealing with only four cells (nations) and one space capsule (Figure 25). In the nervous system we are dealing with billions of cells. Nevertheless, the central nervous system can, to a considerable degree, compensate for loss of lines of communication (nerve cell bodies and all of their processes) by re-routing its information through circuits still left intact. It is only when the damage becomes too extensive that we find nervous system deficit. In this case, the nervous system is no longer capable of compensating for the loss in its lines of communications. How-

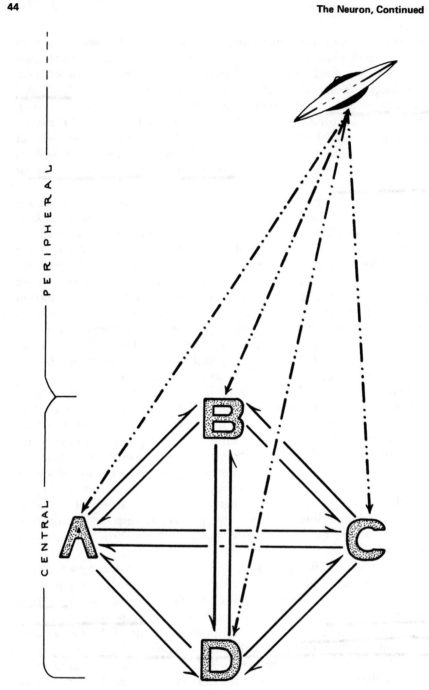

Figure 25.

ever, one can never be sure how severe the damage is until a thorough evaluation has been made and all known measures of rehabilitation have been utilized in an attempt to reeducate or recondition other circuits (the remaining lines of communication) within the nervous system.

Chapter IV

The Neuron (Concluded)

The Location of Cell Bodies in the
Central Nervous System

THE GENERAL LOCATION OF CELL BODIES
IN THE SPINAL CORD

The neuronal cell body is the "battery" for sustaining the life and normal functioning of a neuron (Figure 8, Chapter II). It is important to establish a concept concerning where these cell bodies are located (structural relationships) and how they are arranged into functional components. The first principle to remember is that most neuronal cell bodies are located in an area relatively safe from injury. Usually they are found within or surrounded by a bony covering or deeply embedded in the walls of an organ. No nerve cell bodies are found under the skin or even near its surface. Therefore these very vital yet microscopic bodies are fairly well protected from everyday insult.

The second principle concerns the "color" of the cell bodies that make up the gray areas of the central nervous system (CNS). In the spinal cord there is a central gray area, the *gray matter* (Figure 8, Chapter II). Surrounding this is the *white matter*. In a cross-sectional view of the fresh spinal cord the central area appears pinkish-*gray,* while the surrounding area is pinkish-*white.* What makes this color difference? The central area is gray because this is where the cell bodies of neurons are located. These bodies do not have any covering (myelin or neurolemma sheath) and therefore they are gray in color. The processes (axon and dendrites) extending from them lack a myelin covering also, but once each axon extends beyond the gray area, it obtains its own covering. (Myelin is a lipid-protein material that looks pinkish-white.) Thus, the white matter is white because it is composed of axons which have their own myelin sheaths. A view of a cross-sectional slice of a muskmelon gives the same appearance. Dark tan seeds imbedded in a dark orange pulp (representing cell bodies, dendrites and the beginnings of axons) are located centrally (Figure 26). Surrounding this lies a lighter yellowish-orange area, completely seedless, yet consisting of a very fine fibrous material

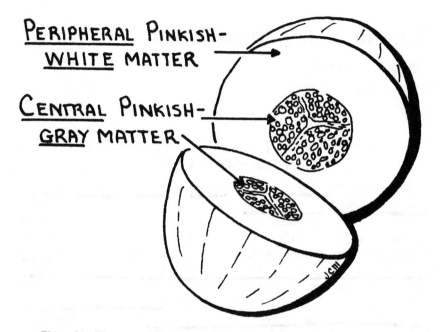

PERIPHERAL PINKISH-
WHITE MATTER

CENTRAL PINKISH-
GRAY MATTER

Figure 26. "Gray and White Matter" of a Muskmelon Simulating the Spinal Cord.

that is compact and yellowish-white. This is analogous to the white matter of the cord or the location of axons.

This simple pattern changes and becomes more complex as progression is made toward higher centers or supraspinal levels. Several exceptions are also found concerning the location of the cell bodies belonging to sensory neurons and those of the autonomic nervous system.

THE LOCATION OF CELL BODIES
OF SENSORY NEURONS

Many of the cell bodies of sensory neurons are located in special places. They still obey the general rule of being protected by, within, or adjacent to a bony protective area or foramen (foramen L.: an aperture or perforation through a bone ... Stedman's). The dorsal root ganglia (ganglion Gr.: an aggregation of nerve cells ... Stedman's) are good examples of these kinds of nerve cell groupings. Each sensory neuron entering the central nervous system has its cell body located just medial to or within the intervertebral foramen (Figure 27 a and b). More explicitly, the peripheral process of each sensory neuron passes through its respective intervertebral foramena and then becomes an enlarged nodule. From this enlargement the central process continues into the "back door" or posterior horn area of the spinal cord (Figure 27c). Careful examination will show that just in front of or ventral to this enlarged area, and incorporated into the fibrous sheath surrounding it, is the motor or ventral root (Figure 27c). Thus, the dorsal root ganglion appears slightly larger, because of the addition of the ventral root so closely applied to the anterior (ventral) aspect of this bulbous mass. Most cranial nerves, carrying sensory impulses, have their ganglia located in or very near various foramena found in the cranial vault or skull. A few have their sensory ganglia within or closely applied to the brain stem and cerebrum.

THE GENERAL LOCATION OF NERVE CELL BODIES WITHIN THE BRAIN STEM, CEREBELLUM, AND THE CEREBRUM

In supraspinal areas of the central nervous system a more complex pattern is found, especially as one rises from the lowest brain stem levels to the cerebral cortex. With evolutional changes over millions of years of nervous system development additional layers of gray (and white) matter have been added. These newer areas are no longer centrally located. Deeply located gray areas still exist and are also surrounded by white areas. However, gray cell masses are also found on the periphery of the brain stem, cerebellum and cerebrum. This third layer, not present in the spinal cord, resembles a bark or cortex covering of the white matter. This can be remembered by equating these centers to the trunk of a tree (Figure 28). Centrally lies the oldest core of the trunk, equivalent to the deep nuclear gray masses. Surrounding this are many rings of lighter wood, equivalent to the white matter. Covering all of this is the bark (cortex) of the tree, synonymous with the peripheral gray matter of the cerebrum, cerebellum, and brain stem. As in a tree where the oldest part is centrally located and the most recent is the peripheral bark, the same general concept can be applied to the central nervous system. Generally, it

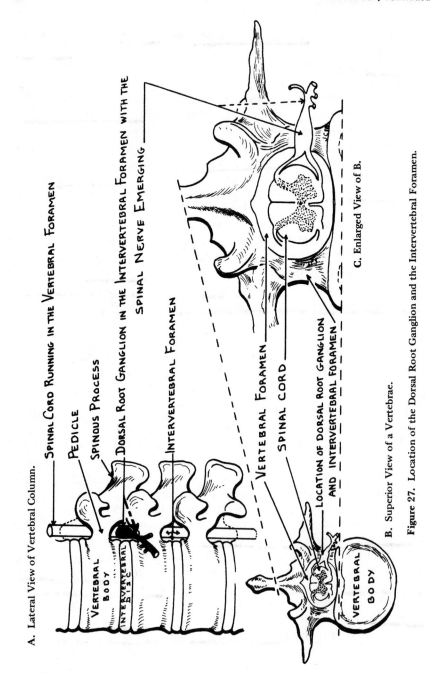

A. Lateral View of Vertebral Column.

B. Superior View of a Vertebrae.

C. Enlarged View of B.

Figure 27. Location of the Dorsal Root Ganglion and the Intervertebral Foramen.

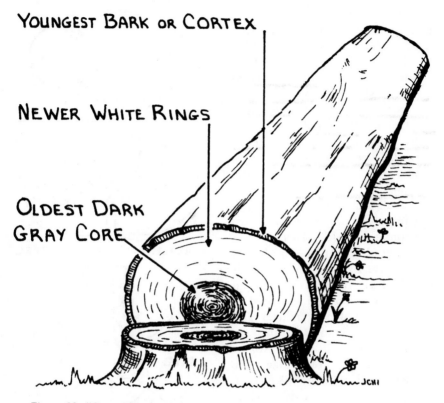

YOUNGEST BARK OR CORTEX

NEWER WHITE RINGS

OLDEST DARK
GRAY CORE

Figure 28. "Gray, White, and Gray Matter" of a tree simulating the Brain Stem, Cerebellum, and Telencephalon.

can be stated that the farther away one goes from the central core, the more recent are the structures whether they belong to the central nervous system or a tree. Similarly, our own nervous system appears to develop from the center outwards. The earliest systems to become functional are the autonomic nervous system and the reticular system, the two most centrally located structures. The last area of man to fully mature is the cerebral cortex, or the most peripherally located structure of the entire CNS.

A CLOSER LOOK AT SPINAL CORD NUCLEI

As previously stated, the nuclei in the spinal cord are centrally located. An "H" or "butterfly pattern" results from the way in which these cell bodies are grouped (Figure 30a). This extremely important central area harbors cell bodies concerned with interneurons and motoneurons having to do with integrating and responding to all three kinds of sensory stimuli (exteroceptive, proprioceptive, and interoceptive). This gray area serves as a reception, processing and redistribution center for impulses coming in (or leaving) over the 31 pairs of spinal nerves, as well as for all ascending and descending impulses passing up or down the spinal cord. (See Part I).

It should be recognized that every level of the spinal cord is somewhat different from all other levels. Constant change in the amount of gray matter and white matter modifies the appearance of each level. Anatomists generally recognize five typical levels (Figure 29). Why does this variation exist? When limb buds first appeared in the development of animals additional cell bodies and their processes were needed to properly control these extremities. Therefore, in the brachial plexus area of the cord (supplying peripheral nerves of the upper limb) and the lumbosacral plexus area (supplying nerves to the lower limb and pelvic area) additional nerve cell bodies were added, especially to the ventrolateral periphery of the central gray area. These new masses of nuclei create a bulge,

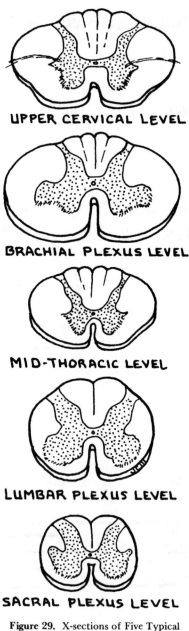

UPPER CERVICAL LEVEL

BRACHIAL PLEXUS LEVEL

MID-THORACIC LEVEL

LUMBAR PLEXUS LEVEL

SACRAL PLEXUS LEVEL

Figure 29. X-sections of Five Typical Spinal Cord Levels.

seen in the ventral horn area, just anteriolateral to the bottom of the "H" (Figure 30b). These areas of the cord look quite different from the upper cervical, or thoracic cord levels, as neither of these two levels makes a major nerve contribution to the limbs. However, another pattern is noticed in the thoracic level where no limb buds exist. Here the butterfly pattern lacks the additional anterolateral gray horn projection. However, cell bodies of the sympathetic division of the autonomic nervous system (ANS) are found at this level as well as at upper lumbar levels (Figure 30c). These cell bodies are readily identifiable as they make a pointed projection of gray matter just opposite or lateral to the cross bar of the "H" pattern. This projection is spoken of as the lateral gray horn. It is strictly for ANS functioning.

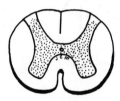

BUTTERFLY OR "H"
PATTERN REPRESENTING
THE GRAY AREA OF THE
SPINAL CORD

A.

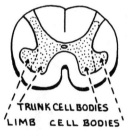

/ TRUNK CELL BODIES \
'LIMB CELL BODIES'

B.

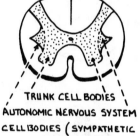

/ TRUNK CELL BODIES \
AUTONOMIC NERVOUS SYSTEM
CELL BODIES (SYMPATHETIC
DIVISION)

C.

Figure 30. Variations in the Butterfly Pattern of the Spinal Cord.

Once these variations in distribution of the gray matter are recognized, then the next step can be taken. The "H" pattern can be divided into its three major components: (1) the dorsal (sensory) gray horns; (2) the centrolateral (ANS) gray horns; and the (3) ventral (motor) gray horns (Figure 31 a and b). Each of these three major divisions can be further subdivided into smaller and smaller, but very important, structural and functional units. Those desiring to study these segments in greater detail may refer to Figures 31c and d. These illustrations give a simple to complex progression of the various areas and their functional importance. Each illustration represents a "composite" cord level, that is, a hypothetical level which does not necessarily exist nor is it truly representative of any one

A. Hypothetical Cross-Section of the Spinal Cord.

B. Three Basic Subdivisions.

DORSAL (SENSORY) GRAY HORN

CENTRAL GRAY AND LATERAL GRAY HORN

VENTRAL (MOTOR) GRAY HORN

C. Functional and Structural Subdivisions.

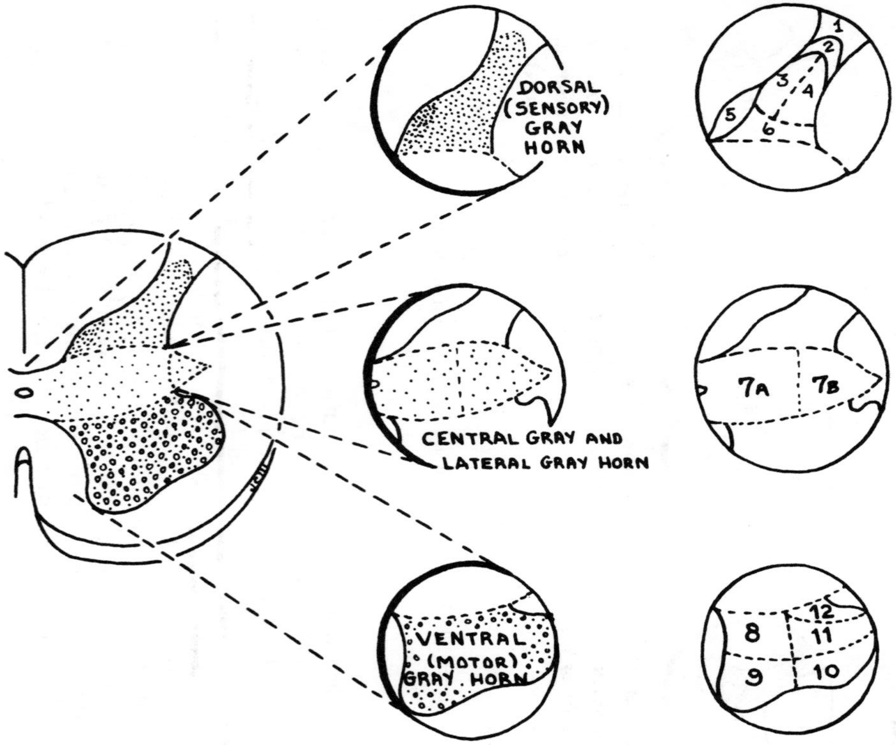

D. Names and General Functions of Subdivisions.

1. LISSAUER'S TRACT: ASCENDING AND DESCENDING COLLATERALS OF PAIN AND TEMPERATURE FIBERS.

2. SUBSTANTIA GELATINOSA: SYNAPTIC AREA FOR PAIN & TEMP. FIBERS

3. DORSAL FUNICULAR GRAY - MEDIAL: SYNAPSES FOR TACTILE & PROPRIOCEPTION

4. DOR. FUNIC. GRAY - LATERAL: SYNAPSES FOR PAIN & TEMP. FIBERS

5. CLARKE'S (DORSAL) NUCLEUS: SYNAPSES FOR UNCON. PROPRIOCEPTION.

6. SECONDARY VISCERAL GRAY: SYNAPTIC AREA FOR AUTONOMIC NERVOUS SYSTEM

7A + B. INTEROMEDIOMEDIAL & INTEROMEDIOLATERAL GRAY: MOTOR CELLS OF SYMPATHETIC DIVISION OF A.N.S

8 & 9. DORSOMEDIAL & VENTROMEDIAL NUCLEI: MOTOR CELL FOR THE NECK, TRUNK, INTERCOSTALS & ABDOMINALS - AT APPROPRIATE LEVELS.

10. VENTROLATERAL NUCLEUS: MOTOR CELLS FOR ARM AND/OR THIGH.

11. DORSOLATERAL NUCLEUS: MOTOR CELLS FOR FOREARM AND/OR LEG.

12. RETRODORSAL NUCLEUS: MOTOR CELLS FOR HANDS AND/OR FEET.

Figure 31. Structural and Functional Divisions of the Gray Matter.

specific cross section. However, this composite serves as a typical pattern for discussing the various parts of the spinal cord gray.

A CLOSER LOOK AT BRAIN STEM NUCLEI

The brain stem is somewhat harder to visualize and understand than is the spinal cord or cerebrum. Numerous changes take place from one level to the next, both structurally and functionally. Name changes add to the confusion. The centers of ten of the 12 cranial nerves are located here. Peduncles (peduncle: little foot, stalk or stem) which are comprised of axons making a variety of connections between the brain stem and the cerebellum are found here (Chapter I, Figure 2). Located in the brain stem are vital centers (respiratory, cardiac, etc.) which govern lower centers and in turn are governed by higher centers. The principle centers of the reticular system also reside throughout this area. New layers have been added during the evolution of these older parts. The white and gray matter is no longer as distinct from one another as was seen at spinal cord levels, but is intermingled or more interdigitated. In spite of these complications and differences a concept can be established in order to gain enough knowledge and familiarity with this vital part of the CNS.

THE HOT DOG BUN ANALOGY

The Hot Dog and Bun analogy will help one to remember this important link between the spinal cord and the cerebrum. Picture a foot-long hot dog nestled between two layers of an eight inch bun (Figure 32a). Notice that the frankfurter extends beyond either end. Consider the lower half of the bun as the basal (anterior or ventral) part of this brain stem model. The wiener represents the central core. The upper part of the bun is the roof (tectum) (Figure 32a). Next artificially divide this sandwich into three parts, as shown in Figure 32b: let both ends of the frankfurter protrude out beyond these three major divisions. The caudal or inferior part of the bun-wiener combination represents the medulla (myelencephalon). Next, is the pons (metencephalon) and last is the midbrain (mesencephalon) (see also Chapter I, Figure 2). That part of the hot dog which protrudes out of the cephalic or far end of the sandwich is the diencephalon.[1]

---

1. Some authors divide the brain stem into three parts (medulla, pons and midbrain). Others consider the diencephalon either as a fourth part of the brain stem, or treat it separately. Throughout this book the brain stem will be considered as having three divisions. The diencephalon will be treated as a separate entity, or as the "through-brain," through which all impulses (except olfaction) must pass before reaching the telencephalon.

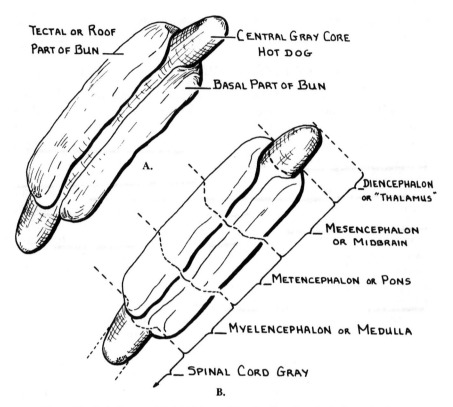

Figure 32. Basic Parts and Subdivisions of the Hot-Dog-Bun Brain Stem Analogy.

That which projects from the caudal or near end represents the up-permost (cervical) levels of the spinal cord gray matter. With our multi-layered-bun-hot-dog combination, we now have three layers (basal, intermediate core, and roof) and three divisions (medulla, pons and midbrain), plus the projecting ends of the wiener demon-strating the continuity of lower and higher parts of the CNS with the brain stem.

The bottom or basal part of this sandwich and the roof represent newer layers added to the older central core. Generally speaking, the basal part consists of express tracts or long pathways (pyramidal tracts) that are newer in development. Included in this area are the more recent nuclear areas (inferior olivary nucleus) directly asso-ciated with some recent gray cell nuclei located in the deeper parts of the cerebellar hemispheres (the dentate nucleus). The roof (tectum) represents recent additions to the central core and could be loosely equated with a bark or cortex for this part of the CNS. The intermediate part represents the old central gray cell body, a direct continuation of the spinal cord gray. However, it should be remembered that in the central core of the brain stem there is no longer a definite separation between gray and white matter. Instead, the gray and white are somewhat intermingled. This can be remembered by inspecting the cross section of any modern day frankfurter. Particles of fat (white matter) are found throughout the meaty substance (gray cell bodies). Thus, the wiener of today very closely resembles the central area of the brain stem. One more concept should be added. This is the correct placement of the ventricular system (cerebral aqueduct, fourth ventricle and central canal carrying cerebral spinal fluid) in relation to the body of the brain stem. When watching individuals put mustard on their wieners, one notices that many people put a thin strip of mustard along the very top surface of the wiener, or between it and the roof of the bun. This is a perfect location as this is the same area in the brain stem where the ventricular system is located (Figure 33). This thin line of mustard (cerebral aqueduct, fourth ventricle, and central canal) acts as a landmark

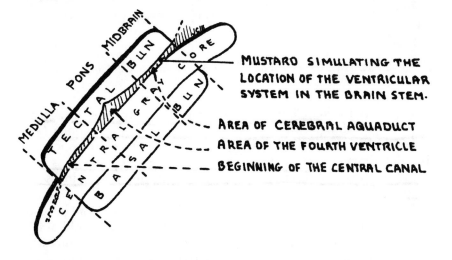

MUSTARD SIMULATING THE
LOCATION OF THE VENTRICULAR
SYSTEM IN THE BRAIN STEM.

AREA OF CEREBRAL AQUADUCT
AREA OF THE FOURTH VENTRICLE
BEGINNING OF THE CENTRAL CANAL

Figure 33. Midsaggittal Section of the Hot-dog-bun.

separating the tectum (roof bun) from the intermediate central core. This mustard analogy enables one to remember that above this landmark lie the newer "cortical centers" of the brain stem, while below it is the central core or oldest area of the brain stem.

In the lowest or medullary division of this sandwich the tectum of the upper medulla can be equated to the archicerebellum, or ancient part of the cerebellum (Figure 34). Even though the archicerebellum is phylogenetically ancient, it is still more recent, developmentally speaking, than the central core of the brain stem. This ancient cere-

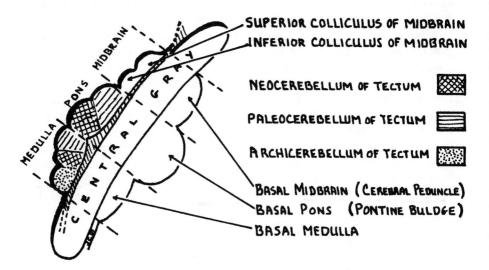

Figure 34. Major Divisions of the Tectal and Basal Areas of the Hot-dog-bun.

bellar area is for stabilizing or balancing the body in space. It developed right along with the vestibular centers of the medulla (vestibular nuclei of the 8th cranial nerve). These areas are concerned with the timing, coordination and smoothing out of actions that depend upon equilibrium or balance of the organism, principally for the trunk.

The roof or tectum of the pons is the paleocerebellum and parts of the neocerebellum (Figure 34) (paleo: second period or old as opposed to archi: first, oldest, or ancient, and neo: new or youngest).[2]

The midbrain tectum is more specialized. It consists in part of the neocerebellum and the two twin bumps (colliculi or little hills) found dorsal to the cerebral aqueduct. These four specialized mounds (two little hills one above the other on each side of the dorsal midline)

---

2. These newer parts developed in higher vertebrates having well developed limbs. Many of the cerebellar nuclei aid in the coordination, stabilization and equilibrium of the limbs in respect to the body.

have been given the following name: the corpora quadrigemini
(body + four + twin). Individually they are spoken of as the
Superior Colliculi (concerned with primitive visual reflexes) and the
Inferior Colliculi (concerned with primitive hearing reflexes).

The neocerebellar part of the tectum developed along with the
appearance of the cerebral cortex. In this way cortical influences
from the cerebrum (telencephalon) can be transmitted directly to the
cerebellum (via corticopontocerebellar tracts or cerebral cortex—
basal pons—neocerebellar route). This enables the cerebellum to continually monitor, smooth out, coordinate and time all actions,
thought processes, and numerous sensations coming in from these
highest centers, with all other parts of the total organism.

As ascent is made from lower to higher levels of the brain stem,
more and more substance is being added to both the roof and the
basal parts (Figure 34). It would be wise at this time to reshape our
visual picture of the hot-dog-bun analogy, tapering the caudal end
and expanding the cephalic end. Add to this a hand, firmly grasping
the central part (Figure 35a). This should enable the reader to conceptualize what the brain stem and cerebellum look like, and have
some idea of its important parts and connections. From this beginning one can correlate the familiar (hot-dog-bun = firmly-grasped-
in-hand) with the less familiar, the brain stem of the central nervous
system. [Figures 36a, b, and c show location, relationship and general function of specific nuclear areas of the brain stem and the
cranial nerve nuclei. These illustrations were adapted from the
Warner-Chilcott[3] brain stem model. This 9-inch model, made out of
a vinyl composition is an excellent aid for understanding the com-
plexities of the brain stem and the diencephalon.]

A CLOSER LOOK AT DIENCEPHALIC NUCLEI

The diencephalon lies between the brain stem and the highest
center of nervous system integration, the telencephalon (tele: distant, encephalon: brain). All sensory impulses reaching the telencephalon (except for olfaction: smell) must pass *through* this area. In
naming this part of the nervous system our forefathers were wise to
call it the *through brain* or diencephalon (dia: through, encephalon:
brain). They recognized its extreme importance as a synaptic center
for sensory stimuli as well as being an integrative center for both
sensory and motor impulses. Though this center is subcortical, recent
research has demonstrated that certain stimuli can be perceived or

---

3. *Vunatomy* by Warner-Chilcott Laboratories, Morris Plains, New Jersey.

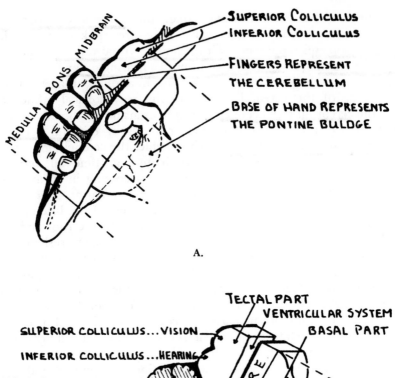

A.

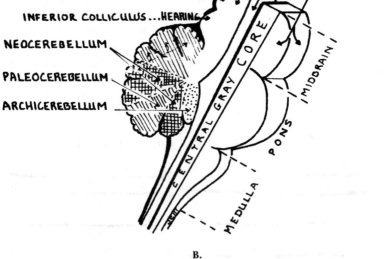

B.

Figure 35. Visualizing the Brain Stem using Simplified Illustrations.

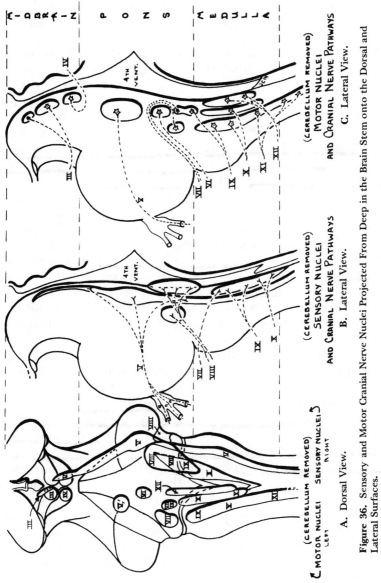

Figure 36. Sensory and Motor Cranial Nerve Nuclei Projected From Deep in the Brain Stem onto the Dorsal and Lateral Surfaces.

A. Dorsal View.

B. Lateral View.

C. Lateral View.

vaguely recognized at this level. Previously it was believed that only those impulses reaching the cerebral cortex were the ones which the organism could feel or understand.

In our hot-dog-bun analogy the cephalic end of the hot dog purposely protruded out beyond the bun. It was stated that this projecting part represented the diencephalon. And well it does, as the diencephalon is practically an all gray area, made up of numerous cell body clusters, each having a specialized function. All clusters are intimately interconnected with surrounding areas of the CNS. Actually, five rather distinct divisions of the diencephalon are recognized: (1) dorsal thalamus, (2) hypothalamus, (3) sub or ventral thalamus, (4) epithalamus and (5) the metathalamus. Notice that the term thalamus is the common name for all five of these areas. The adjective or prefix preceding this term merely tells the reader which part is being discussed, its location, and possibly its function. In other words, the dorsal thalamus lies somewhat dorsal in the area of the diencephalon. The hypothalamus lies *below* this. The *meta*thalamus *beyond* it (actually posterio-inferior to the dorsal thalamus). The epithalamus lies *above* or is uppermost in the diencephalon. The *sub* (or ventral) thalamus lies in the lowest part. This is no different from naming the floors of a building as a sub-basement, first floor, mezzanine, top floor, etc.

It is interesting to note the derivation of the word thalamus (a word many people use either as a synonym for the diencephalon, or more commonly for the *dorsal thalamus*). The Latin word *thalamus* (from the Greek thalamos) means "a bridal chamber." The diencephalon is centrally located in the deepest part of the brain, almost as if it were a hidden or very private room. It is surrounded above and medially by the ventricular system, and laterally and inferiorly by masses of white tracts (making up part of the internal capsule) that carry impulses into and out of this chamber room (Figure 37a and b). Why does such a small area, interposed between the brain stem and the telencephalon, have such an important role, and what are some of the more important functions of these deep nuclear gray masses? To explain these questions, only three of the five nuclear centers will be discussed: (1) the dorsal thalamus (2) the metathalamus and (3) the hypothalamus.

The major function of the dorsal thalamus is to act as a receiving and sending station for all sensory input (except olfaction) going to consciousness. So far as is known, every impulse must synapse here before it can continue to higher centers. In other words, the dorsal thalamus acts as a redistribution center for impulses coming in from

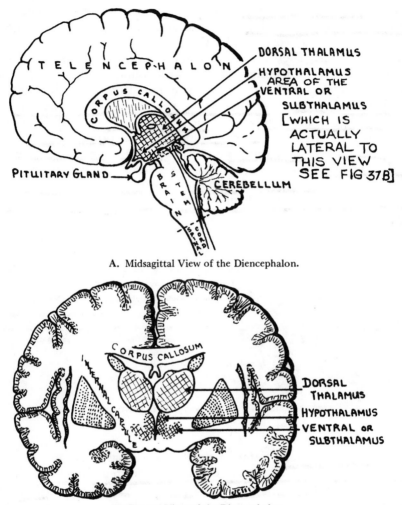

A. Midsagittal View of the Diencephalon.

B. Frontal View of the Diencephalon.

Figure 37. Diencephalic Area = Cross Hatched.
Basal Ganglia Area = Dotted.

peripheral nerves, spinal cord levels, brain stem nuclei, the cerebellum and, from the cranial nerves. Undoubtedly all this sensory
information is integrated and refined here, as well as being compared
with all other information being received, including impulses from
the telencephalon itself. Therefore, all impulses passing to the cerebral cortex are made much more meaningful because of this process
of evaluation continually taking place in the dorsal thalamus.

The metathalamus consists of two rounded nuclear masses, the medial and lateral geniculate (L. genu: knee) bodies. These two knee-like bumps are tucked up under the posterior-inferior aspect of the dorsal thalamus. They are directly related to, and intimately connected with the two bumps or little hills found on the dorsum (or tectal area) of the midbrain, the superior and inferior colliculi. As the inferior colliculi are a primitive receptive and reflex auditory center, the medial geniculate body is the diencephalic center for this kind of sensation. Likewise, the superior colliculi are the primitive centers of the midbrain for visual reflexes, and the lateral geniculate nucleus is its diencephalic center (Figure 38). These two genicular masses are responsible for evaluating, integrating and finally distributing visual and auditory impulses to higher centers of the central nervous system.

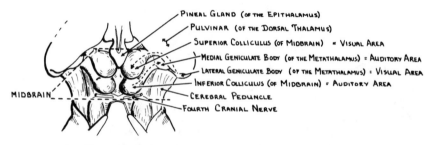

Figure 38. Dorsal View of the Midbrain and Metathalamus.

The hypothalamus, found beneath the dorsal thalamus, is the master controller of all autonomic nervous system functions. It is concerned with emotional states and feelings of well-being or general malaise and is intricately interconnected with the frontal lobes of the cerebral cortex, the limbic lobe system, reticular system, pituitary gland, brain stem nuclei, basal ganglion, *et al.* (Figure 39).

A CLOSER LOOK AT TELENCEPHALIC NUCLEI

Like the spinal cord, brain stem or cerebellum, the telencephalon has a central gray area surrounded by white matter. But unlike the spinal cord it has a mantel of peripherally located gray matter, the many-layered cerebral cortex. The central gray area is the basal ganglia, a collection of specialized nuclei (ganglia) surrounding the dien-

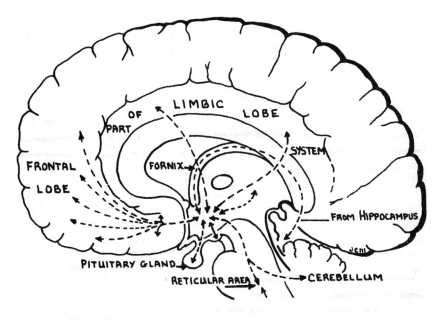

Figure 39. Connections to and from the Hypothalamus—Schematic.

cephalon and located near the base of the brain. One might equate this part of the CNS with the rings of a tree that has grown somewhat lopsided over millions of years of drought (gray matter) and plenty (white matter) (Figure 40). Notice the repeated patterns of gray, white, gray, white and finally gray. Complexity results when all the developmental flexures, curvatures and infoldings (convolutions) are added to this simple concept. However, slight modification of the tree ring illustration (Figure 41) gives a fairly close resemblance to the frontal view of the major parts of the telencephalon which

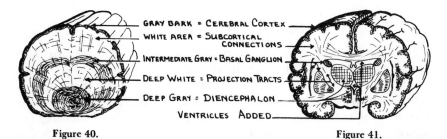

GRAY BARK = CEREBRAL CORTEX
WHITE AREA = SUBCORTICAL CONNECTIONS
INTERMEDIATE GRAY = BASAL GANGLION
DEEP WHITE = PROJECTION TRACTS
DEEP GRAY = DIENCEPHALON
VENTRICLES ADDED

Figure 40.   Figure 41.

Figure 40-41. Lopsided Tree Rings Simulating the Frontal Section of the Brain.

surround the diencephalon (Figure 37a and 41). Notice in Figure 41 that the lateral ventricles and the third ventricle have been added to give their proper relationship to this graphic illustration. The peripheral cortex is purposely kept thin to simulate the extremely narrow mantel of gray (1 to 4 mm average thickness) that covers our brains.

What can be stated for the general functions of these two additional gray areas, the basal ganglia and the cerebral cortex? The basal ganglia can be considered as the highest facilitory and inhibitory sensorimotor area concerned with governing stereotyped or automatic reflexes. The automatic arm swing in rhythm with walking is just one of many examples that can be cited. Well documented animal behavioral studies have demonstrated how uniform these basic patterns are in all species of animals (including man) and how they continually act as a background of purposeful movement and behavior in every aspect of life. The basal ganglia as well as other subcortical areas is also believed to be the major storage center for "learned reflexes" (or semiautomatic reflexes) such as writing, dressing, eating, walking, typing, etc.

The telencephalic cerebral cortex, the very highest sensorimotor center, is believed to be responsible for our ability to learn how to act, communicate and associate past events with present ones. It enables man to recognize sensations and/or associate two or more past events in order to create new situations, ideas or learned behavioral patterns. It is this area of the nervous system that takes the longest to fully develop or mature (twenty plus years). It is this area that man depends upon for his successes or failures in our modern day society. Its many layers appear to be highly specialized (though less so than originally believed) for receiving, processing and integrating stimuli reaching these levels from subcortical areas. Without it, man is virtually helpless; yet it in turn depends totally upon all other parts of the nervous system and the body as a whole in order to function in a meaningful and purposeful manner.

THE "C" SHAPE CONCEPT

The highest centers of the nervous system are not very easy to understand even with the simple analogies just presented. A reason for this may be the fact that one must first develop a three-dimensional concept before being able to visualize the various structures found in the cerebrum. Many of the important parts of this area are highly curved like a "C" lying on its side " ⌒ ". Such structures as the lateral ventricles, the limbic lobe complex, the fornix-hippocampal systems, caudate nucleus, corpus callosum, and even the cerebral cortex itself all conform to the side-lying "C" pattern (Figure 42a, b, c, and d). How can one remember that these structures are tightly curved?

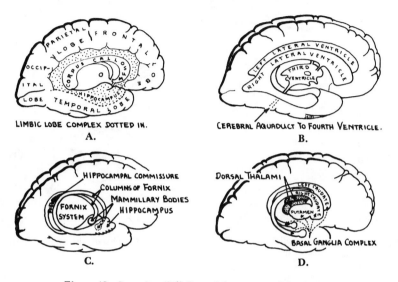

Figure 42. Curved or "C" Shaped Structures of the Brain.

One might answer this by postulating that during the millions of years of evolutionary changes the brain continued to grow and expand in some areas and at the same time modify old parts for newer purposes. During this growth period the brain remained relatively confined within the very slowly expanding and ever changing dimensions of the bony vault. The best possible way to conform to a circular or curved vault structure is to curl up into a "C" pattern utilizing the entire area instead of leaving dead spaces. Also, the addition of more and more convolutions (gyri and sulci, or hills and valleys) gave the brain greater surface area, yet maintained the total brain within the limits of the gradually changing protective skull.

Our own two hands are the best tools we have for visualizing and understanding these three dimensional curved structures of the brain (Figure 43). Picture the thumb side of the hand as the lateral aspect of one cerebral hemisphere, the little finger side as the mid-sagittal plane or medial aspect of that same hemisphere. In lower animals the brain appears "flattened" or stretched out, as your hand would be in

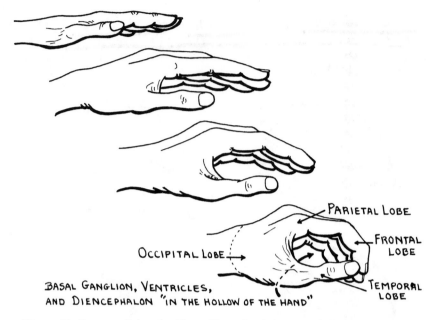

PARIETAL LOBE

FRONTAL LOBE

OCCIPITAL LOBE→

BASAL GANGLION, VENTRICLES, AND DIENCEPHALON "IN THE HOLLOW OF THE HAND"

TEMPORAL LOBE

Figure 43. Conceptualizing the Three Dimensional Aspects of the Brain and the Curved Structures within it.

full extension. As the phylogenetic scale is ascended the brain appears to take on a greater curvature similar to a slightly flexed hand. Man's brain appears like the cupped hand in Figure 43. In changing the hand from full extension to the naturally flexed position, notice that the thumb moves outward and into abduction. This places the thumb somewhat laterally with respect to the curved fingers and simulates the position of the temporal lobe in relation to the frontal, parietal and occipital lobes that are represented by the fingers and body of the hand. Imagine that the dorsal skin represents the cerebral cortex. The muscles, tendons, vessels, and bone represent the various curved structures mentioned earlier (corpus callosum, limbic lobe system, caudate nucleus, etc.) as well as the white tracts found beneath the gray mantel. Thus, all of these deeper structures take on the curved position, making it easier to see how these various nuclear masses assumed this shape. Into the hollow of the hand one may now place the cephalic end of the hot dog, the diencephalon. The space surrounding the diencephalon represents the ventricular system. To complete the picture place both hands together with the little fingers adjacent to one another. Cross your forearms to accomplish this. In this way one can simulate the entire curved brain (both cerebral hemispheres) within the cranial vault. The diencephalon fills the hollow of the hands and the brain stem protrudes dorsally and inferiorly from this area.

SUMMARY

The general location and importance of the gray nuclear areas in the spinal cord, brain stem and cerebellum, diencephalon, and telencephalon have been presented. Similarities and differences between the lowest parts of the CNS and the highest, with gradual changes taking place as one ascends the brain stem and reaches diencephalic levels, have been stressed. Emphasis has been placed upon these nuclear areas because this is where the "batteries of neurons," or their cell bodies, are found. The specific interconnecting wires (white matter or tracts) to and from these batteries tying the central, peripheral, and autonomic nervous systems into one functioning unit have purposefully been omitted. Once understanding as to the location of these functional nuclear areas is achieved, then the highways and byways (wires or neuronal processes) can be added. This approach is akin to learning geography. It is much easier to memorize the general placement of towns, cities, and countries than it is to learn concurrently every road leading into or out of each area, or even to know the boundaries and relative positions of one nation to another. It is hoped that the analogies put forth (hot-dog-bun, hands simulating the telencephalon, etc.) will enable the reader to have a better grasp of the nervous system and to visualize how each part fits together into a structural and functional whole.

Chapter V

A New Look at the Nervous System in Relation to Rehabilitation Techniques

INTRODUCTION

In order to discuss new concepts relating to the nervous system, one needs a yardstick against which to measure changes. This yardstick is the information found in our older textbooks. Many of the "newer" undergraduate texts (1965 to 1968 publications) still hold to older ideas concerning nervous system functioning. Only the more recent ones, usually written on the graduate level, attempt to bring the reader up to date. Unfortunately, these newer texts are not being utilized as much as they should be. This is probably because of the depth of information within them, especially as regards recent research findings in neuroanatomy, neurophysiology, psychobiology, etc.

Another yardstick which can be used concerns the amount of knowledge the average therapist should have in order to adequately treat patients and converse with associates. This yardstick can only be applied to those therapists desiring more information in the area of neurobiology. Perhaps the best measure can be found in the number of workshops, special classes, lectures, *et al.*, that have been and are being offered every year on this subject. The fact that a more-than-adequate attendance is usually found at these events is evidence in itself. Coupled with this is the knowledge that today approximately 50 per cent of all of the case loads, in any given hospital or clinic, consists of patients having neurological involvement. Therefore, it would appear that at least an "adequate" knowledge is a necessary pre-requisite for all therapists. For those involved in the teaching and training of therapists, a *more than* adequate knowledge is, of course, necessary.

What is an adequate knowledge? First, it should be up-to-date information. Second, it should give the therapist enough vocabulary, morphology, physiology, and understanding so that he can talk intelligently with his associates. Third, it should enable the therapist to begin to understand and/or explain to some degree what they are attempting to accomplish in therapy.

It also means "unlearning" earlier concepts or theories previously taught as fact. This automatically implies new learning and new understanding. At the same time one must realize that today's knowledge may become out-dated (to varying degrees) within a year or more after it is learned. This is due to the vast amount of research being published today in the neurosciences. These very important papers are beginning to help therapists explain what they are doing in treatment.

What then are some of the old concepts we once learned which today need to be up-dated? How do these more recent ideas help us understand some of our treatment techniques?

MOTOR AND SENSORY

In the past the emphasis was on the motor side of nervous system functioning. This seemed reasonable. This side is readily seen, measured and manipulated. It is the easiest part of the nervous system to remember because it is so apparent. In the past, we gave voice to the sensory side, but only secondarily. Most individuals can remember the pyramidal tracts and their functions. How many can recall fasciculus cuneatus, dorsal spinocerebellar tract, ventral spinothalamic tract, etc., not to speak of their functions? Or to express it in the most obvious way: the motor side was thought to be simple in comparison to the sensory side which is extremely complex.

Researchers have spent a lifetime studying only one sensory organ (such as the eye, ear, skin, etc.). We still are far from understanding everything about even the simplest of receptors. The motor side was thought to have been understood "years ago." Just three main components were believed to have been involved: (1) the pyramidal tracts, (2) the extrapyramidal tracts, and (3) the final common pathway or lower motoneuron, now called the alpha motoneuron. We thought we had this "motor side" pretty well understood when we catagorized these three motor components into neat "memory packages." See Table 1.

There are no compact "memory charts" for the sensory side of the nervous system, unless one desires to become ridiculous and catagorize the senses as in Table 2.

TABLE 1

	Pyramidal Tracts	Extrapyramidal Tracts	Lower (LMN) Motoneurons
Speed:	Fastest tracts	Slower tracts	Faster tracts
Synapses:	One synapse	Many synapses	No synapses, direct to myoneural junction.
Age:	Recent	Old	Probably new (unknown)
Origin:	Area 4 (pre-central gyrus or motor strip)	Basal ganglia and midbrain	Ventral horn cell
Termination:	Directly on LMN	Directly to LMN	Muscle
Controls:	Opposite side of body	Both sides of body	One side of body with contralateral effects
Function:	Fine, coordinative	Gross movements	Muscle contraction
Lesion:	Flaccidity (rarely see)	Spasticity (commonly see, in all degrees)	Flaccidity and degeneration

TABLE 2

Sensors	Functions
Eyes	Sight
Ears	Hearing
Tongue	Taste
Nose	Smell
Labyrinth	Balance
Joints, tendons, etc.	Movement monitors
Skin	Feelings
Etc.	Etc.

Such a chart fails to tell us HOW we see, feel, hear or act. Also, neither chart even begins to let us understand HOW the nervous system functions in integrating these senses in order to obtain a response. A huge abyss exists in our ability to bridge the chasm of knowledge between motor and sensory. Not only this, but we have "learned" the nervous system backwards, putting the cart before the horse. We think, talk and act in a frame of reference that is MOTOR-SENSORY.

What if we "unlearned" our previous knowledge and began thinking in reverse, i.e., SENSORY-MOTOR! Thinking this way would automatically accomplish two things: First, we would become more acutely aware of all of the sensations we are putting into a nervous system during treatment; second, we should begin to wonder how these sensations interact and cause the nervous system to respond. Just as an example (to illustrate how ingrained our minds have become in our reversed learning and thinking) a recent and very valuable publication still appears to emphasize motor over sensory.[1] Such phrases as "motor learning," "motor behavior," "neuromotor pathology" etc., are used throughout this book.

Until we reverse our thinking, our teaching and our way of looking at the nervous system, we may never understand how it functions, or why a patient responds as he does to various stimuli around him.

PYRAMIDAL AND EXTRAPYRAMIDAL SYSTEMS

In the past, writers catagorized the nervous system into discreet entities in order to better understand it. An example is the PYRA-MIDAL SYSTEM. Actually this term only implies an anatomical definition. Neurophysiologically it fails to help us understand how this tract functions. Another system or category was the EXTRA-PYRAMIDAL SYSTEM. Again, this term is only an anatomical definition and does not help us understand function. Also this term is no longer acceptable in regard to more recent neurophysiological research. Rather it handicaps us in our ability to comprehend how things work.

Does a pyramidal system exist? Yes, there are pyramidal tracts. It has always been stated that these tracts originated in Area 4 (the precentral gyrus or motor strip of the cerebral cortex). However, today we know that only about 40 per cent of the fibers of this pyramidal system originate from this area. Other areas include the postcentral gyrus (Areas 3, 1, and 2, or the sensory strip of the cerebral cortex) and the adjacent parietal and frontal lobes, the occipital lobes and some from the temporal lobe. Thus 40 to 60 per cent come from Areas 3, 1, 2, and 4, the primary sensory and motor corticies. The remaining fibers come from the rest of the cerebral cortex.[2]

These fibers converge and descend through the internal capsule to reach the medullary pyramids of the lower medulla. Here in the "pyramidal decussation" 70 to 90 per cent cross over to the contra-lateral side and form the lateral corticospinal tract. The rest descend on the ipsilateral side as the ventral corticospinal tract. However, more recent evidence tells us that the majority of fibers originating in the cerebral cortex as "pyramidal tract fibers" never reach the med-ullary pyramids. Instead, many of them terminate in the pons where they synapse with pontocerebellar tracts. These tracts cross over to the contralateral neocerebellum (the phylogenetically youngest areas of the cerebellum). They inform the cerebellum about the impulses initiated in the cerebral cortex. A direct feedback from neocerebellar nuclei (dentate nucleus) to the cortex (via dentothalamocortical tracts and dentorubrospinal tracts) also exists.[2,3] Thus the cerebellum can act as an almost instantaneous monitor and integrator (or synchronizer) upon the descending pyramidal tracts (Figure 44).

Therefore, few pyramidal tract fibers actually originate from just Area 4. Few ever reach the medullary pyramids (whence these tracts derived their name) and few ever reach lower motoneurons. Many of those which eventually reach lower motoneurons only do so indirectly, as we shall see later. Therefore, our old anatomical definition of the pyramidal system appears to be vague, doubtful, and perhaps quite misleading. Modern writers are pleading that this term be eliminated from our neuroanatomical and neurophysiological vocabulary.[2-6] It should be, as it no longer helps explain how the nervous system functions. Rather, it is misleading. It channels our minds into accepting false doctrines of nervous system integration and function, especially as regards pathological conditions which we deal with clinically.

How about the extrapyramidal system? Does the anatomical definition of this system still hold true today? We learned that this system had its origin in the basal ganglion and the midbrain (and some lower levels of the brain stem if we include the reticular formation in the over-all definition). Today we know differently. The extrapyramidal system is now spoken of as "coeps," meaning the cortically originating extra-pyramidal system.[2] Like the pyramidal system it also originates from Areas 4, 3, 1 and 2, and other areas of the frontal, parietal, temporal and occipital lobes, as well as the insula and rhinencephalon. Granted it is an older system than the more recent pyramidal system but are the differences between these two systems as great as we once assumed? Both originate in similar areas of the cerebral cortex. Both have numerous connections with the cerebellum, basal ganglia, reticular formation and other brain stem nuclei. Both influence lower motoneurons. No longer is the pyramidal system considered as just a two-neuron chain in contrast to the extrapyramidal system. Both are polysynaptic (multisynaptic), the extrapyramidal system only being more so. Both tracts may be able to influence a motoneuron at approximately the same given time, in spite of synaptic delays and varying conduction velocities. In fact the pyramidal system may not be able to act at all until the

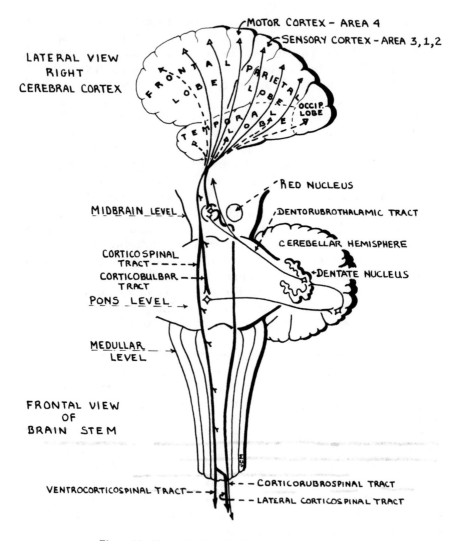

Figure 44. "Pyramidal Tract" Origins and Connections.

extrapyramidal system and other influencing stimuli have set the
stage (or threshold) upon which the pyramidal system can act. Therefore, it would be wise for modern day therapists to eliminate these
old terms and ideas so firmly fixed in their minds and begin to think
in terms of specific pathways, their connections, and how these interact to produce desired movement.

THE RETICULAR SYSTEM

This term stems from the word "net" or "network." During early research on the nervous system definitive tracts and nuclear groups which were readily discernible (with the aid of the microscope) were identified and defined. In the brain stem, after discreet nuclei and tracts were accounted for, there remained several large, yet loosely connected, areas of unknown function. These were difficult to categorize. Their cell bodies were of all sizes and their fiber connections were extremely numerous and complex. These areas became known as the reticular formation of the brain stem, a network of loosely connected nuclei and fiber systems running through the medulla, pons and the midbrain (Figure 45).

Later work showed that this area was important in keeping the organism awake and alert. Also evidence indicated that it had a decided influence over lower motoneurons. It was learned still later that almost all other areas of the nervous system (both sensory and motor) fed information into this system. More recently this area has lost its confinement to just the brain-stem levels. It is known to extend throughout all segments of the spinal cord and continues through the diencephalon.[2][6] It also has extensive connections with the cerebellum as well as the cerebral cortex and basal ganglion. (Figures 45 and 46).

Phylogenetically it is perhaps the oldest entity of the nervous system. Yet as old as it is, we are far from realizing the full extent of this system's function, especially as regards its interactions with other areas of the nervous system. Diffuse as it may be, it does have definite inhibitory and facilitory effects upon motoneurons controlling our actions and behavior. It also appears to be responsible for our state of awareness, our degree of alertness, and our ability to stay awake for sixteen or more hours a day.

THE RUBROSPINAL TRACT

This small tract (Figure 47) once thought to be non-existent or insignificant in man (but more important in lower animals) is making a comeback today. It was once said that if it existed in man, it originated from the red nucleus of the midbrain, and descended only as far as cervical cord levels. It was known to have connections with the cerebellum via the dentrorubrospinal tract (Figure 47). It was classified as one of the many extrapyramidal tracts, and was believed to have exerted its influence only upon structures of the head and

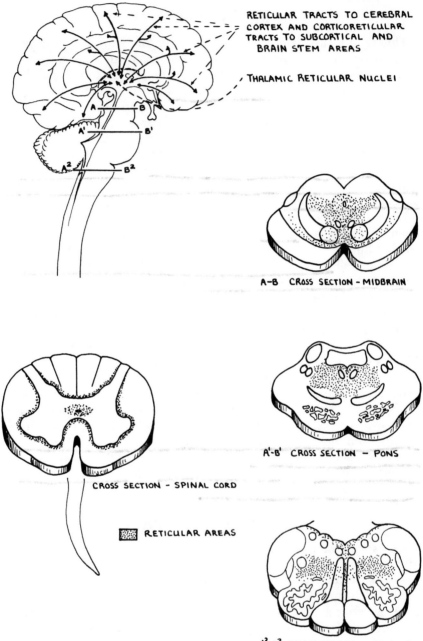

RETICULAR TRACTS TO CEREBRAL CORTEX AND CORTICORETICULAR TRACTS TO SUBCORTICAL AND BRAIN STEM AREAS

THALAMIC RETICULAR NUCLEI

A-B CROSS SECTION - MIDBRAIN

A'-B' CROSS SECTION - PONS

CROSS SECTION - SPINAL CORD

RETICULAR AREAS

A²-B² CROSS SECTION - MEDULLA

Figure 45. Reticular Areas of the Central Nervous System.

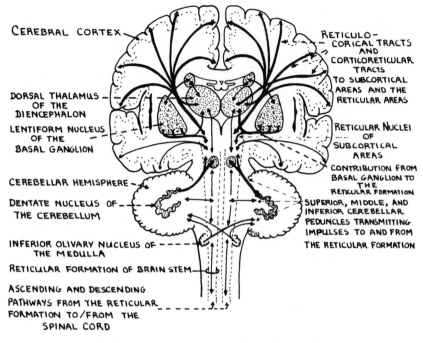

CEREBRAL CORTEX

RETICULO-CORICAL TRACTS AND CORTICORETICULAR TRACTS TO SUBCORTICAL AREAS AND THE RETICULAR AREAS

DORSAL THALAMUS OF THE DIENCEPHALON

LENTIFORM NUCLEUS OF THE BASAL GANGLION

RETICULAR NUCLEI OF SUBCORTICAL AREAS

CEREBELLAR HEMISPHERE

DENTATE NUCLEUS OF THE CEREBELLUM

CONTRIBUTION FROM BASAL GANGLION TO THE RETICULAR FORMATION

SUPERIOR, MIDDLE, AND INFERIOR CEREBELLAR PEDUNCLES TRANSMITTING IMPULSES TO AND FROM THE RETICULAR FORMATION

INFERIOR OLIVARY NUCLEUS OF THE MEDULLA

RETICULAR FORMATION OF BRAIN STEM

ASCENDING AND DESCENDING PATHWAYS FROM THE RETICULAR FORMATION TO/FROM THE SPINAL CORD

Figure 46. Some Connections of the Reticular System (Schematic).

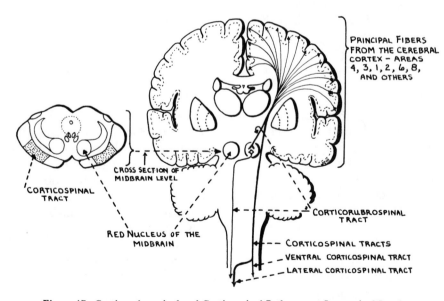

PRINCIPAL FIBERS FROM THE CEREBRAL CORTEX — AREAS 4, 3, 1, 2, 6, 8, AND OTHERS

CROSS SECTION OF MIDBRAIN LEVEL

CORTICOSPINAL TRACT

CORTICORUBROSPINAL TRACT

CORTICOSPINAL TRACTS
VENTRAL CORTICOSPINAL TRACT
LATERAL CORTICOSPINAL TRACT

RED NUCLEUS OF THE MIDBRAIN

Figure 47. Corticorubrospinal and Corticospinal Pathways at Supraspinal Levels.

neck. New evidence brings this tract into more meaningful perspective. For one, it probably originates at cortical levels as witnessed by its modern name, corticorubrospinal tract. Two, it may function as a partner, or companion, of the lateral corticospinal tract (Figure 48). Three, it is now known to extend down as far as and including lumbar levels of the spinal cord. Thus it has influence over many more levels of the body musculature than originally supposed.

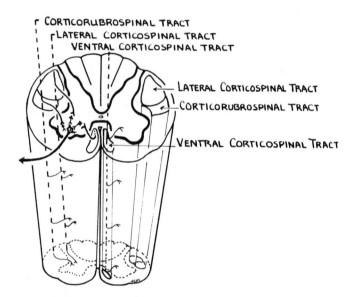

Figure 48. Corticospinal and Corticorubrospinal Pathways at Spinal Cord Levels.

Recent research indicates that this tract (as well as the corticospinal tract) is probably facilitory to flexors (adductors and internal rotators) and inhibitory to extensors (abductors and external rotators). (Figure 49) Hence we see two tracts working together, the lateral corticospinal tract (a pyramidal tract) and the corticorubrospinal tract (an extrapyramidal tract). Both tracts share extensive connections with the cerebellum, basal ganglia and midbrain. Both appear to be very important to nervous system functioning.

Many other tracts could be mentioned, but these few serve as the principle examples of how our concepts of nervous system functioning are indeed changing. It is these changes which are beginning to

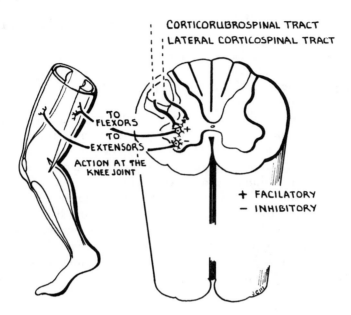

Figure 49. Facilitory and Inhibitory Influences Via Corticospinal and Corticorubrospinal Tracts.

add that necessary degree of knowledge which is so vital for understanding nervous system pathology and treatment.

VENTRAL GRAY HORN NUCLEI

Many years ago our teaching centered around the large ventral horn (motor) cells of the nervous system. These cells were supposed to be responsible for all movement and were called the final common pathway or the lower motoneuron. Descending tracts and reflex connections were thought to synapse directly onto these ventral horn cells in order to cause coordinated movement.

In the past few decades, however, several other kinds of ventral horn cells have been recognized. Each appears to have a different individualistic function. Some are, indeed, our old friends the ventral horn cells (now called the alpha motoneuron). However, many others exist. Some are believed to be only inhibitory, others only excitatory to the alpha motoneuron. Renshaw cells, beta (?) cells, and certainly gamma cells are also found in this ventral horn gray area. Many interneurons and recurrent collateral fibers are also recognized. The

ventral gray area has become a complex zone and a heaven for researchers. All is not understood nor agreed upon as yet for these
numerous kinds of cells. However, from the voluminous research
literature being published, several concepts are emerging which can
give us some ideas as to how this area functions in expressing the
organisms response to stimuli.

We are fairly certain of the location of flexor (adductor and internal rotator) and extensor (abductor and external rotator) motoneurons of the alpha variety. (Figure 50a) The gamma motoneurons,
having to do with these same functional groups, are probably located
in and around the alpha motoneurons. The same appears to be true
for the other kinds of cells noted. Some interneurons are located in
the dorsal gray horn, others in the ventral horn, and still others cross
over to the contralateral ventral horn area. Recurrent collaterals
(branches from alpha motoneurons) recur, or feedback, in the ventral
horn cell areas whence they came and synapse on interneurons of the
Renshaw variety (Figure 50b).

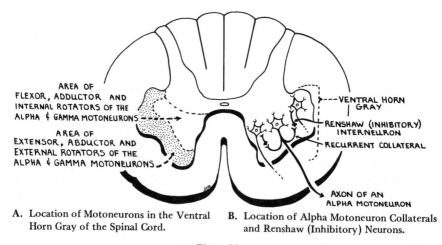

A. Location of Motoneurons in the Ventral   B. Location of Alpha Motoneuron Collaterals
   Horn Gray of the Spinal Cord.   and Renshaw (Inhibitory) Neurons.

Figure 50.

What are the functional implications of these numerous cell types?
Many are tonically inhibitory or excitatory to motoneurons, i.e.,
they help change the threshold of cells upon which they synapse.
Thus a given motoneuron cannot fire (or can fire readily) according
to the demands of the stimuli presented to the organism. Others
prevent a reverberating circuit such as is seen in clonus. Renshaw
cells (which are interneurons of a certain variety) are specifically

inhibitory to motoneurons upon which they synapse. Alpha motoneurons are equivalent to our old lower motoneurons, or the final
common pathway. However, the concepts governing the alpha motoneuron's ability to fire (send impulses) is gravely different from what
was once thought. Gamma motoneurons have become the center of
attention in their ability and importance in controlling muscle function.

GAMMA AND ALPHA MOTONEURONS

The gamma motoneuron (so named because this type of cell is
much smaller than the largest ventral horn cell or alpha motoneuron)
is now believed to be the main route or circuit through which almost
all of the descending pathways travel (Figure 51). We once thought
that almost everything (ascending, descending and reflex circuits)
synapsed directly upon the alpha motonueron. Now we know that
this is not true. We are fairly certain that the majority of our reflex
pathways used during normal activities of daily living, probably
synapse upon the gamma motoneurons first and only indirectly upon
the alphas (Figure 48-51).

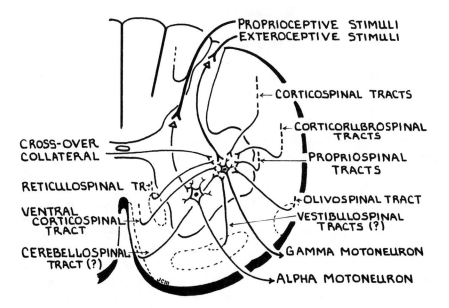

Figure 51. Some synapses on the gamma motoneuron.

(Certain exceptions probably exist, but as yet there is no general agreement about this. Examples may be one of the vestibulospinal tracts and those fibers of the lateral corticospinal tract which go to alpha motoneurons supplying the muscles of the hands and feet.)

What is the purpose of such a circuitous route, this gamma loop system, or in a broader manner of speaking, the alpha-gamma linkage system? Why use the gamma loop system first before ever getting the impulse to the alpha motoneuron? The alpha motoneuron is, after all, the final neuron which enables skeletal muscles to contract!

On the surface it would appear as if nature has interposed an extra delay into the nervous system, one that might slow down our actions instead of speeding them up. However, one must keep in mind the fact that man is not, and never has been, a very speedy organism. In relation to most other mammals, man is extremely slow when all factors are considered. However, he probably has the most complicated nervous system known. His dependence for survival and communal living vary greatly from others in the animal kingdom. His ability to exist and function depends more upon the capacity to learn, communicate, remember and interpret the total environment than upon speed, skill, strength, stereotyped reflexes or instinct. Thus man needs complex sensors which will continually relate him to his total environment. This must be monitored in such a way that the human is constantly aware (either cortically or subcortically) of every action or change in both the external surroundings and his internal environment.

The gamma loop system, as well as many other feedback circuits built into our nervous systems, provides all of these important sensors. It acts as judge of every change made within or without the organism. Like the eyes, cochlea, vestibular apparatus, etc., it alerts and prepares the organism to any change about to take place, taking place, or having taken place. It is a past, present, and future monitor of the final expression of man's total being, i.e., movement. Without this, man ceases to function normally. In primitive times he did not survive. However, with this sensor system—(1) the gamma motoneuron, (2) the neuromuscular and neurotendinous spindles and other motion sensors, (3) the afferent feedback route to the alpha motoneurons and to many other nerve centers—it becomes the principle regulator of all action or non-action (Figure 52). It can facilitate or inhibit motion. Through it the cerebral cortex (and all other centers concerned with motion) can exert their influences so that coordinated and purposeful movement can be obtained in response to all stimuli having any influence upon the organism at any given

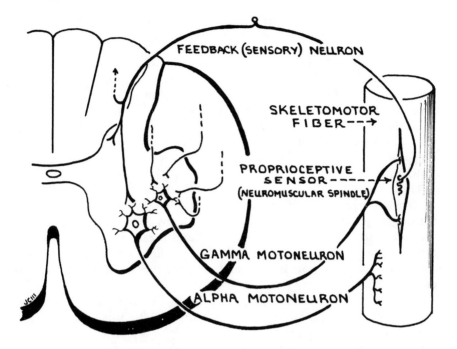

FEEDBACK (SENSORY) NEURON

SKELETOMOTOR FIBER--→

PROPRIOCEPTIVE SENSOR-----→
(NEUROMUSCULAR SPINDLE)

GAMMA MOTONEURON

ALPHA MOTONEURON

Figure 52. The Alpha-Gamma Linkage System.

moment. Fortunately this gamma loop sensor system can also be manipulated by outside influences such as pressure, stretch, temperature, balance, touch, etc. Thus we have ways of influencing this all-important part of the nervous system by manipulating it and making it purposefully act upon the rest of the nervous system.

The alpha motoneuron, once thought to be the most important cell body governing motion, is now subjucated to some extent by the gamma system. In spite of this, the alpha motoneuron is still extremely important. Without it normal movement may not take place in the skeletal muscle fibers it supplies. However, it appears to be subservient to all other parts of the nervous system with some possible exceptions.[5] It cannot function by itself until its threshold has been properly set by numerous other influences impinging upon it, including the gamma loop system. Destroy some of the inhibitory and facilitory influences regulating its threshold and one destroys the ability of this motoneuron to carry out normal movement patterns, even though it has not, of itself, been diseased or injured in any way.

THE NEUROMUSCULAR SPINDLE
(INTRAFUSAL OR FUSIMOTOR FIBER)

A few years ago we thought we had some of the answers concerning the function of the neuromuscular spindle. Today we find no general agreement, other than the fact it is probably a length and tension receptor for skeletomotor fibers.[4,5,7-10] Until more research is forthcoming, we are just about where we started five or more years ago. However, it is generally agreed that this "length and tension receptor" can act in at least two ways in order to influence muscular function.

(1) It can regulate, via supraspinal influences, the amount of tone or tension which will be necessary in skeletomotor fibers, for any action about to take place. This is done by supraspinal pathways synapsing on the gamma motoneuron and presetting or biasing the muscle spindle. In turn, changes in the spindle send impulses to the alpha-motoneuron, which fires and changes the tension of the skeletomotor fibers.

(2) The neuromuscular spindle of itself, by constantly recording the amount of length and/or tension in the skeletomotor fibers (once movement has taken place) can influence the alpha motoneuron as well as the rest of the nervous system. We shall have to wait for more concrete evidence before we can definitely state what the other function(s) are of this extremely complex receptor, i.e., its precise facilitory and inhibitory effects on skeletomotor fibers. About the same can be said for the function of the neurotendinous spindle. We know that these receptors have facilitory and inhibitory actions but exactly what this is, or how it works is as yet quite unsettled.

However, some other new and interesting facts have recently appeared concerning the neuromuscular spindle. This concerns the population density of these spindle receptors in skeletomotor (extrafusal) fibers. From the meager evidence we presently have[4,5,7-10] it appears that the highest concentration of spindles is found in the deep cervical neck muscles. The next highest, in the intrinsic muscles of the hands and feet(the interossei, lumbricales, et al.) The ribs (intercostals) appear to have the next highest concentration.

So far we have dealt with muscles that are concerned with fine, coordinative, regulatory or manipulative actions of the body. These muscles are very small and delicate compared to such muscles as the triceps, trapezius, soleus, glutei. As one grades over from the fine delicate musculature to the more proximal trunk and girdle muscles one appears to find fewer and fewer spindles per skeletomotor muscle mass.

(Unfortunately, very little is known about the spindle populations of muscles innervated by cranial nerves, such as muscles of facial expression, chewing, swallowing, phonation, hearing, orbital muscles and the like. When these facts come to light, we can speculate that spindle populations in these will be extremely dense. This supposition is based on the fact that these skeletomotor fibers are responsible for fine delicate control and coordination of some of our most important sensorimotor systems of the body).

If one begins to analyze spindle density in light of growth and development, a new concept seems to emerge. Those areas of the body most necessary for survival and for exploring the environment (in order to become oriented in it so that one may then become acquainted with it and thus learn from it) are the areas with the apparently highest spindle population. Certainly the neck righting reflexes (which are intricately associated with the vestibular and optic righting reflexes) are all important to the infant's ability to orient his head, and then his body, in space so that he may eventually roll over, crawl, creep and finally free his hands for cruising, walking and exploring his universe. Through his hands and feet he constantly explores his limited environment, bringing objects closer to his visual and auditory fields as well as his most highly developed areas, his lips, mouth and tongue.[11/13]

The importance of the high spindle population in the deep neck muscles cannot be minimized. Many of the so-called "extrapyramidal" tracts have long been known to reach only cervical levels. Perhaps they need not descend any further. We have known from experiments on lower animals and on man that the neck reflexes (asymetrical and symetrical) govern the actions of the upper limbs, hence the trunk, and finally the lower-limb musculature. Research on normal adults has proven and re-proven that these tonic neck reflexes still influence our everyday actions by causing tonus changes in our upper-limb musculature as the head is rotated, flexed or extended.

As adults we know that our most skilled movements are performed by such muscles as the lumbricales, interossei, thenar and hypothenar muscles. As more information is published, undoubtedly the muscles of the vocal apparatus, the orbit, or the ear will also be added to the list of muscles having high spindle populations.

If one watches the developing infant, growing into the child and eventually the adult, one notices that these very areas of high spindle density are perhaps the last areas of the total body musculature to fully develop to their highest functional degree. The infant's cry is gross in comparison to the adult opera singer. The facial musculature gives generalized smiles or frowns (almost stereotyped) compared to the fine control of facial expression and communication used between adults. The baby's head is wobbly on his "rubbery" neck for many months. Fine control of head movement does not appear until much later. The hands are the last to achieve their final manipulative skill.

Could we conceptualize and postulate that the greater the spindle population, the longer it takes for this musculature to mature (keeping in mind at all times the cephalo-caudal law of development, whereby the more cephalic levels of the body mature earlier than the more distal or caudal)? Could we go one step further and reason that maturity of body musculature may be directly dependent upon spindle density and hence the alpha-gamma linkage system?

It would appear, from the slim evidence we now have, that the higher the spindle density (and thus the greater the number of alpha-gamma linkages) the longer it takes to learn to control these muscles and eventually use them to their maximum. Therefore those muscles with the lowest spindle population should be the easiest to rehabilitate (girdle and trunk musculature). Those in the intermediate-density range (arm, thigh, and leg muscles) should be the next easiest. The hardest to rehabilitate, as we have known for years, are the deep neck muscles and those of the forearm, hands and feet. Inability to gain control of this high spindle density musculature leaves the patient unable to control or orient his head (and all of its very vital senses) in space. Likewise, inability to gain control of his distal limb musculature leaves the patient severely handicapped in his ability to function in society. It is interesting to note that in old age palsies, and in Parkinson's disease, these areas of apparently high spindle populations are the earliest ones affected.

This theory in no way implies that one should begin rehabilitating distal musculature over proximal ones. Rather the cephalo-caudal law of development should be held to, whereby therapy is begun in those areas which are known to develop first, the lips, mouth and tongue, followed by the neck, proximal trunk and girdle muscles, etc.[11/13] Also before fine control can be gained over the intrinsic cervical muscles the most gross neck muscles (superficial musculature having lower spindle density) should be rehabilitated first.

Granted this theory is based in part upon neurophysiological research, but it is also based upon clinical observation. At the moment it would appear to be meaningful in light of our newer exteroceptive and proprioceptive rehabilitation techniques. What is more, perhaps for the first time we have a more workable hypothesis on which to base treatment techniques. Knowingly or not, we have been rehabilitating low spindle density musculature and cephalic areas before attempting intermediate or high-density musculature, and thus more caudal or distal areas.

PLASTICITY AND LEARNING IN THE NERVOUS SYSTEM

How does the nervous system learn? Nobody really knows for sure. However, scientists have presented a number of creditable theories on this subject. This is an area in which rehabilitationists should be keenly interested. After all, rehabilitation or habilitation is a means of "teaching a nervous system" how to perform slightly differently, or in a new way, so that it can better react to, or cope with, its environment. What are some of these more recent concepts? How might these ideas be useful to those using the newer rehabilitation techniques?

It is still believed that when we are born we possess our full compliment of neurons. Approximately twenty billion neurons exist in the brain,[3] not to mention other areas of the nervous system. This in no way implies that the nervous system is "mature" at birth. Far from it. It only means that we cannot gain additional neurons during life, or replace damaged or lost ones. However, we know that the nervous system matures slowly over a period of eighteen to twenty-one years or longer.[11/13] This means that other properties of the nervous system are constantly changing as growth, development, learning and memory take place.

What are these "changing" or "maturing" factors that enable the nervous system to become more complex and skilled as the years advance? To date research has shown that changes are constantly taking place in the following structures: (1) dendritic growth, (2) an increase in myelination of neuronal processes, (3) changes at or within synapses and the changing of synapses, (4) collateral growth of axons, (5) new end-plate development, (6) growth of new receptor cells replacing old or damaged ones in some systems of the body, and (7) the use of different or less-used neuronal circuits.

These factors and many more can be cited as evidence for a plastic nervous system. In some respects this nervous system never ceases changing or maturing yet in some other aspects it probably reaches its fullest maturity in the second or third decade of life. All of these factors have a direct bearing upon how the nervous system learns, matures, remembers and communicates.

Were the nervous system a rigid, non-plastic, unchangeable structure at birth, no learning would occur. Rather, like very low forms of life we would operate by pure instinct with stereotyped reflexes. However, we know that the nervous system learns, and in so doing, constantly changes. From experiments on rats, it has been shown that a "super-environment" (extra handling, good exercise, etc.) increases the gram weight of their brains compared to controls.[3] A deprived environment retards the animal and slows down growth and development. We have seen this same effect on man, but we needed experiments on rats to show how these factors affected the nervous system.

Likewise the brain-injured lower animal, if allowed to exercise and receive a good diet, will make a remarkable recovery to the extent that his nervous system deficit is recognized only by the trained observer.[5] In rehabilitation we see patients learn to compensate for nervous system deficits and find new ways in which they can function in their environment. Were the nervous system not pliable, rehabilitation would be purposeless.

It would appear that a direct correlation exists between a plastic nervous system and (1) the environment, (2) growth and development, and (3) learning (Figure 53). Take away any one of these three components and the organism fails to mature and/or survive. Without stimuli or with insufficient stimuli it cannot function or develop normally. It may not even be able to learn. All three entities are INTERdependent to the normal functioning of this pliable nervous system. It would also appear that the nervous system is, initially, entirely dependent upon purposeful stimuli (imput) in order to help it develop and begin to learn. Likewise, the ability of the system to learn depends upon purposeful output. The stimulus has to be *meaningful* in order for the system to respond and remember the stimulus. Use abnormal input or deprive the organism of stimuli and one sees abnormal output, and eventually nervous system degeneration.

Cerebral palsied children are excellent examples of nervous systems with abnormal input. Many are incapable of seeing, hearing, balancing or moving in a purposeful manner. Thus the input from their environment is interpreted by their receptors and the central nervous system, as faulty. Complicating this is the feedback from these purposeless responses into an already damaged nervous system. This system has just responded to these stimuli by using faulty receptors. Now it is even more confused by this feedback from purposeless output. How can it begin to make sense out of all of these purposeless stimuli constantly bombarding it? More and more ab-

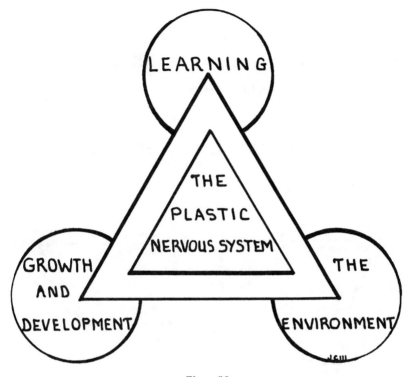

Figure 53.

normal input results in more purposeless output.[14] A vicious cycle results (Figure 54).

No wonder this damaged nervous system is handicapped in its ability to mature, learn, remember and respond purposefully. Each repetition of the cycle (Figure 54) accentuates the pattern until movement is stopped or complete frustration results. Then a new hit-or-miss approach is attempted by the organism which is still trying to make some sense out of the environment. One way in which the nervous system copes with this problem is to tighten up or become semirigid. This lessens faulty feedback from meaningless movement patterns in response to the various stimuli. It may also enable the organism to respond to less and less stimuli around it. Thus if the receptors can respond to fewer stimuli, and perhaps in a more purposeful manner, some of the exaggerated faulty feedback can be eliminated. The system may then be able to make more sense out of the stimuli constantly influencing it.

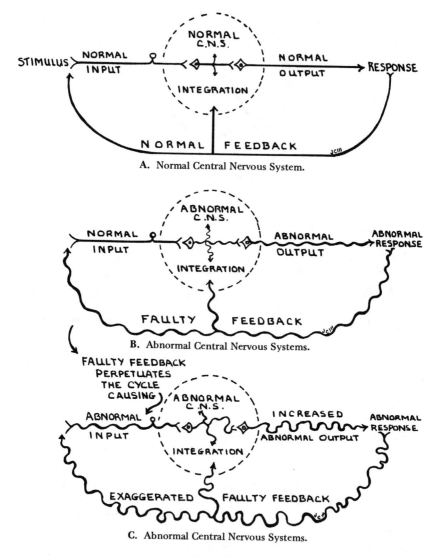

A. Normal Central Nervous System.

B. Abnormal Central Nervous Systems.

C. Abnormal Central Nervous Systems.

Figure 54.

Braces, added weights, restraints and the like, have been man's attempt to do this for the cerebral palsied child. These measures attempted to cut down or help eliminate purposeless input by harnessing the areas most severely involved. This was intended to break the cycle of purposeless input ⟶ poor integration ⟶ purposeless output ⟶ exaggerated faulty feedback. In accomplishing this, it may also have resulted in producing a rigid, non-plastic nervous system at a much earlier age than we see in the normal.

What are some other concepts concerning nervous system learning and plasticity? How long for instance does it take to learn to write? Not one of us can remember. We have forgotten the number of times we repeated, over and over again, certain letters, words, and finally phrases in order to perfect our writing ability. Whether it took one year or five years to progress from meaningless scribbling to printing and finally writing, is not important. What is important is that it was an extremely long time, and a very tedious process.

How about changing hand dominance?* If as normal adults we were to change handedness, we could be guaranteed that it would take over a year before one would have to stop saying to himself, "Oh, I'm supposed to use the other hand." It will take over ten years before it becomes a subcortical response.

What is meant by this term subcortical? Suppose we attempt changing dominance every day, constantly. We begin by doing it on a cortical or completely conscious level. Every movement or act is noted by the individual! Every error is noted as frustration or the inability to change dominance and smooth out the intricate actions involved.

During the first several years of practice all actions are accomplished by tightening up, or becoming tense, while trying to control the muscles of the once non-dominant hand. It is not until we consciously begin to relax, take everything more slowly, precisely and gently, do we begin to succeed in our efforts. However, with repeated efforts, and after about ten years of more of intense, yet relaxed practice, the actions finally become automatic, that is, subcortical. This means that we no longer have to remind ourselves to switch hands when reaching for an object, while eating, dressing, writing, etc. It is accomplished without tenseness and done so smoothly that the nervous system is no longer consciously aware that the action is taking place.

If one were to switch hand dominance in the older child, it could be accomplished in much less time.[11] If done on the young child just as, or prior to, establishing hand dominance, it can be readily accomplished without the youngster being aware of it.[11] This is because it is accomplished on a completely subcortical level and on a very plastic and immature nervous system. The youngster is not aware of

---

*This term in no way implies "brain dominance." Rather it refers only to the dominant hand, i.e., right- or left-handedness.

it even though the trainer or parent is. The infant is "learning" by mimicking the actions of others. No conscious thought is involved. In fact, his cortical areas are not as yet developed sufficiently to use them for conscious learning.[11,13]

Learning on the subcortical level is believed to be much faster than attempting it on the cortical (conscious) level. As we get older, and our nervous system matures at higher and higher levels, we lose a certain ability to learn subcortically. Our systems becomes less and less plastic and our movements become more and more ingrained. Also, we become more conscious of our environment and our actions in response to it. This in no way implies that we lose (until senility) the ability to learn. However, it does become more difficult with advancing age. Collateral growth of axons, dendritic branching, myelination, synaptic changes, *et al.,* still can come about, but much more slowly.[11]

Practically all of the learning we did in infancy and early childhood, such as dressing, feeding, walking, running, drinking, playing, was done on a subcortical level. Initially our mothers and fathers dressed us, fed us, helped us stand, and walked with us. Hundreds of hours were spent by them putting a head through a hole in a sweater, or tucking an arm through a sleeve, or plunging food into our mouths so that we might swallow it. During this time we paid little attention to the activities about us, responding only if hurt, happy or hungry.

Thousands of times the adult made purposeful movements for us, until one day we began doing these things ourselves. First it was on a trial and error basis, crudely attempted and with no real conscious effort involved. Were one to ask the normal child, during this stage of development, to perform an activity like dressing, (before the child had learned it thoroughly) he would become "spastic" trying to accomplish this task. Not spastic as we see it clinically, but a degree of tension and ineptness resembling non-purposeful movement would be seen in this child's actions. However, if the child is allowed to do it without being watched, amazingly enough he accomplishes the task, in his own way, quite well. The difference here is that of trying a task on a cortical level (being asked and being watched usually causes cortical reactions) versus doing it automatically on the subcortical level.

Most of our early learning was on this subcortical level. We copied, even though we did not really know what we were doing, but the results were pleasing to ourselves or to those around us. Therefore repetition of an act won favor and thus reinforcement of that act. However, we did not think about it, we just mimicked what we saw. One day these very actions become ingrained (subcortical) without much cortical involvement ever having taken place.

From studies on the nervous system, it would appear that the subcortical areas (especially the reticular formation) "learn" much faster and more easily than the cerebral cortex. In other words, those areas related to consciousness (which are also the areas of the nervous system that are the most recent in development) are the areas where learning is the slowest, the most difficult, and even sometimes utterly impossible. Sad this is, for in our society today our greatest dependence is on these very areas. However, it is believed that the phylogenetically older systems develop first, "learn faster," and have control over subcortical movements. The newer areas develop last, are slow to "learn" and are believed to be responsible for our control of fine purposeful discriminative movements.

Also, the newer systems appear to be less plastic. They seemingly have fewer alternate pathways, fewer neurons and synapses, and therefore they may be more difficult to influence or change. The older areas of the system appear to be more pliable. They have numerous and multiple connections and pathways. They are capable of carrying out fine enough movements to enable an organism to get along in its environment.

Many of the newer rehabilitation techniques are based upon this concept of subcortical learning. The older techniques were based upon cortical efforts. With the evidence we now have it would appear that subcortical learning is faster, easier, less frustrating and more lasting than cortical learning. Likewise, we have long known that things learned in childhood, whether actions or pieces of information, are the last to be forgotten, or lost, in nervous system disease, injury or senility. Recent (cortical) memory fades quickly and easily.

We have also known that in nervous system damage and recovery, those areas which recover last (or never regain normal function) are those which are phylogenetically younger, or more recent in evolution. Could this also relate in part to spindle density? Those areas which have the highest spindle population may well be the phylogenetically most recent areas to develop. They are the most difficult to initially learn to control, and thus are the most easily affected in nervous system deficit. Therefore, should they not be the hardest areas to regain control over, or to rehabilitate?

EXCITATION, INHIBITION,
AND THE "RELEASE PHENOMENON"

Another fairly new concept of nervous system development should be considered here. It has been postulated that during the earliest functioning of the growing nervous system, excitatory areas develop first. Thus the organism can, up until a certain state, be considered as an excitatory complex. Many of the early inborn reflexes appear to substantiate this theory, such as the fetal grasp reflex, early swimming and walking reflexes, and the Babinski reflex. As growth and development proceeds, and as higher and higher centers of nervous system control mature, inhibitory influences are laid down. These appear to dampen, or over-ride, the older excitatory areas and prevent them from freely expressing themselves. Primitive reflexes are inhibited or greatly diminished in character. They are not seen again unless the organism is damaged. With complete maturation, a fine balance is finally established between these two opposing systems. Thus excitatory centers may be more primitive (phylogenetically older) than the more recent inhibitory centers.

Once central nervous system damage occurs, this delicate balance is upset. Usually this releases older excitatory areas which are no longer held in control by the newer inhibitory centers. The resultant is usually expressed as an excitatory type of behavior: spasticity, rigidity, clonus, tremors, ballism, athetosis, flexor contractures, Babinski reflexes, incoordination, etc. This is sometimes spoken of as a "release phenomenon." The damaged area of the system, in effect, releases all of the other areas which once relayed impulses to it. Now these released centers are "free" to exert their influences (or impulses) upon other centers. This would be equivalent to an army about to attack a town. Upon learning that the town has capitulated, it is free to turn its energies upon other centers (not prepared for this assault) and exert its influences accordingly. In other words, the balance appears to be upset in favor of the phylogenetically older or more primitive excitatory systems.

CONCLUSION

The newer rehabilitation concepts and treatment techniques are attempting to put these new theories of nervous system development and functioning into practice. Therapists are trying to inhibit these "released excitatory centers" by using various exteroceptive and proprioceptive stimuli which can influence the developing and plastic nervous system. They are working at subcortical levels in their attempts to retrain the nervous system. They are using purposeful stimuli by utilizing certain postures and motions which can both inhibit unwanted actions and facilitate desired and meaningful movement. They have based these techniques upon evidence relating to phylogenetic development of the nervous system. They realize that they will never be able to completely rehabilitate a damaged nervous system, especially those areas which are phylogenetically recent. However, clinical evidence is demonstrating that control of input, especially on a subcortical level, can help control output and hence lessen faulty feedback. Repetition of these techniques, day after day, is producing results.

As therapists constantly update their knowledge of treatment techniques, they should also update their knowledge of how the nervous system functions. In understanding these newer concepts we may yet find the answers to our oft repeated questions: Why does nervous system damage cause certain kinds of functional loss? How do these rehabilitation techniques actually affect the maturing nervous system? Are today's techniques better than yesterday's, and if so, how are we going to prove it?

Everyday we are coming closer and closer to some of the answers. However, we must attempt to keep up with the changing concepts coming out of research in the neurosciences, if we ever hope to be ready to understand the answers when they are finally presented to us.

REFERENCES

1. An Exploratory and Analytical Survey of Therapeutic Exercise," Northwestern Univ. Spec. Therapeutic Exercise Project, *Amer J Phys Med*, Wm. & Wilkins Co., 46, 1 (Feb. 1967).
2. Ruch, Patton, Woodbury and Towe, "Neurophysiology," W.B. Saunders Co. (1965).
3. Noback, Chas. R., "The Human Nervous System," McGraw-Hill Pub. Co. (1967).
4. Eccles, Sir J.C., "Functional Organization of the Spinal Cord," *Anesthesiology*, 28, 1 (Jan.-Feb., 1967).
5. Eldred, Earl and Buchwald, Jennifer, "Central Nervous System: Motor Mechanisms," *Ann Rev Phys*, 29, 573-606 (1967).
6. Laursen, A. Mosfeldt, "Higher Functions of the Central Nervous System," *Ann Rev Phys*, 29, 543-572 (1967).
7. Andrew, B.L. (Ed.), "Control and Innervation of Skeletal Muscle." A symposium at Queen's College, Dundee, 1965. Wm. & Wilkins Co. (1966).
8. Bishop, P.O., "Central Nervous System: Afferent Mechanisms and Perception," *Ann Rev Phys*, 29, 427-484 (1967).
9. Granit, R. (Ed.), "Nobel Symposium I. Muscular Afferents and Motor Control," John Wiley & Sons (1966).

10. Granit, R., Kellerth, J., and Szumski, A., "Intracellular Recording from Extensor Motoneurons Activated Across the Gamma Loop," *J Neurophysiol,* 29, 530-544 (1966).
11. Bakes, Frank P., "Speech, Language and Hearing," *In Human Development,* 433-458, Ed. by F. Falkner, W.B. Saunders (1966).
12. Larroche, Jeanne-Caudie, "The Development of the Central Nervous System During Intra-uterine Life: Part II," *In Human Development,* 257-276, Ed. by F. Falkner, W.B. Saunders (1966).
13. Peiper, Albrecht, "Cerebral Function in Infancy and Childhood," *International Behavioral Science Series,* Consultants Bureau, N.Y., p. 683 (1963).
14. Dinnerstein, A.J. and Lowenthal, M., "Teaching Demonstrations of Simulated Disability," *Arch Phys Med,* 49, 3, 167-169 (1968).